INFERTILITIES

CULTURAL STUDIES OF THE AMERICAS

Edited by George Yúdice, Jean Franco, and Juan Flores

Volume 4 *Infertilities: Exploring Fictions of Barren Bodies*
Robin Truth Goodman

Volume 3 *Latin Americanism*
Román de la Campa

Volume 2 *Disidentifications: Queers of Color and the Performance of Politics*
José Esteban Muñoz

Volume 1 *The Fence and the River: Culture and Politics at the U.S.–Mexico Border*
Claire F. Fox

INFERTILITIES

Exploring Fictions of Barren Bodies

Robin Truth Goodman

Cultural Studies of the Americas

VOLUME 4

University of Minnesota Press
Minneapolis
London

Portions of "Conrad's Closet" originally appeared as "Conrad's Closet," *Conradiana* 30, no. 2 (summer 1998): 83–124; published by Texas Tech University Press and reprinted by permission. Portions of "Mario Vargas Llosa and the Rape of Sebastiana" originally appeared as "Mario Vargas Llosa and the Rape of Sebastiana," *Latin American Literary Review* 27, no. 53 (July 1999): 86–107; reprinted by permission of the publisher, *Latin American Literary Review.*

Published by the University of Minnesota Press
111 Third Avenue South, Suite 290
Minneapolis, MN 55401-2520
http://www.upress.umn.edu

Library of Congress Cataloging-in-Publication Data

Goodman, Robin Truth, 1966–
Infertilities: exploring fictions of barren bodies/Robin Truth Goodman.
p. cm.—(Cultural studies of the Americas ; v. 4)
Includes bibliographical references (p.) and index.
ISBN 0-8166-3487-4 (alk. paper)—ISBN 0-8166-3488-2 (pbk. : alk. paper)
1. Spanish American fiction—History and criticism. 2. Conrad, Joseph, 1857–1924—Criticism and interpretation. 3. Infertility, Female, in literature. I. Title. II. Series.
PQ7082.F35 G63 2000
863.009′353—dc21
00-009089

Printed in the United States of America on acid-free paper

11 10 09 08 07 06 05 04 03 02 01 10 9 8 7 6 5 4 3 2 1

Contents

Preface

This book analyzes literary and political representations of female infertility from the mid-nineteenth century to the present. It takes as a starting point Darwin's studies on sterility between species. Darwinian evolutionary science imagines class struggle as a sexual game, recreating colonial history and the struggle for resources within representations of nonreproductive female identities. I trace Darwin's findings through discussions of cultural representations wherein female unreproductiveness is a defining feature, arguing how femininity has come to represent global markets. As such, this book is vitally concerned with the role of the family in policing identity but also with how the family itself is involved—within literature, discourse, and politics—as a defense against the ravages of new capitalist orders. It shows, for example, how Latin America offers an origin story of migrant identities where femininity defines the border along which economic interests—or, rather, the so-called natural freedoms of market enterprise—are seen urgently, like the family, as needing protection. In exploring these issues I examine how Joseph Conrad constructs a vision of feminism as a product of miscegenation, how Alejo Carpentier deploys female homosexuality to figure Latin American literature as difference, and how ecological devastation in the Brazilian Amazon is envisioned as failure in a Native American marriage. By locating points of conjunction between queer, feminist, and postcolonial theories, I trace the ways that evolutionary theory still affects how unreproductive femininity functions within narratives of colonial and postcolonial histories; consequently, I read lesbian and reproductive theory and politics as participating in critiques of globalization.

Although the focus here is mainly on the textual and symbolic fabrics of female infertility—on unraveling, for example, the politics of representation in literature, film, anthropology, theory, and science—I cannot think such issues outside of the political environments that make them important in the contemporary political setting. As Nancy Fraser has pointed out, the current idea of the welfare state is organized on the basis of single-earner households that "provided the normative picture of a proper family" (41). The prevalence of this type of family arrangement was overestimated even during the Industrial Revolution and the beginnings of the welfare state. However, now, in an era of globalization, the family cannot any longer be thought of as the root principle on which economic policy is structured. Even as it is caused by capital shifts and mobility, the coming apart of the family enters culture as a moral problem, usually about women. The current foregrounding of debates about, say, gay and lesbian rights, abortion, or maternal surrogacy brings out female infertility as a hidden thematic setting the tone of much political movement and debate in the United States today. This shows a large amount of cultural anxiety forming around issues of inheritance even as paternity is becoming more ascertainable. This concern with inheritance testifies to a growing insecurity about economic issues more generally, a feeling of instability and panic among ordinary people about the changing nature of industrial production, the limits to social mobility, and the related transformations in workforce roles. Concurrently, the highly politicized dismantling of the welfare system finds justification in images of single, black, poor women who are hyperreproductive and—like the tenement immigrant women identified as eugenic targets for a birth control campaign at the turn of the century—needing financial restrictions on birthing rates. A current distrust or even vilification of sex on the internet has turned into a discussion about the post-human, an apocalyptic vision of a future with babies produced in laboratories (dystopically popularized in the images of human farms in *The Matrix*), while a prevalent belief that unreproductive women are dangerous infiltrates even medical practices—as, I have been warned, turning thirty without ever having been pregnant places me at greater risk for cancer, and, as nurse practitioners have informed me, I should start considering marriage. Such highly volatile, politicized images certainly require dismemberment, and new findings in queer theory are one good place to begin taking them apart.

In addition, much mainstream filmmaking involves plots about the suspension of female reproduction leading to the end of the human as we know it. Human bodies and consciousness are colonized either by technologies and media (e.g., in *Videodrome, Robocop, Total Recall*) or alien invaders (e.g., in *Alien, The Faculty*). Such movies show female sexuality as a place that, apocalyptically, endangers the human. *Independence Day*, for example, starts with the president's wife being called away from her family for personal business on a distant coast. The subsequent weakening of the president's masculinity underpins the global catastrophe of evil aliens crossing into national airspace and the destruction that follows, including the destruction of the First Lady's reproductive capacity through an abdominal injury leading to her death. As much as narratives about universal extinction stigmatize female fertility as a problem, they also show femininity constituted as a site of death, destruction, and danger within, for example, anxious fantasies posing immigration as a threat to national interests. The evil aliens have, after all, come to earth forcefully and unstoppably to take control and ownership of our scarce natural resources. This inalienable hunger of the alien for what is our property and our heritage is intertwined with the First Lady's symbolic abortion, the potential end of the line of our first children. "We are fighting," says the president, prepping his troops for an air raid, "for the right to life." His wife's absence from the scene of reproduction becomes, in a sense, a stand-in plot for an alien conquest, a robbing and removal of our territory. The president can then regain the loss of national economic supremacy only by an excessive show of military violence that reinstates the family—the daughter's love and safety—as the prize of global victory. In other words, the idea of the human that depends on the reproduction of femininity is formed as a grid of global economic power.

One wonders, indeed, if the cultural construction of homosexuality as a problem is essentially, perhaps inextricably, connected to the depiction of the immigrant as a site of panic. "Especially at those junctures," notes Judith Butler, "in which compulsory heterosexuality works in the service of maintaining hegemonic forms of racial purity, the 'threat' of homosexuality takes on a distinctive complexity" (1993: 18). Who, then, benefits as a result of such representations, which merge heteronormativity into injunctions to police national borders? In what sense are served the interests of national labor, the protection of jobs and wage ceilings, the profit of capital, the growth of industry, the credibility of government through such defensive insertions of the family, a return to reproduction at moments of perceived crisis? Such a connection has a history, and this history is necessarily rooted in a conception of feminine identities invented through a science deeply interwoven with the pursuit of empire, the spread of markets, the accumulation of goods, the furtherance of power, and the dawn of globalization.

Acknowledgments

I owe many thanks to George Yúdice who, with his intellectual guidance and faith, helped bring this project to completion, and also to Jean Franco, and to Douglas Armato and Gretchen Asmussen of the University of Minnesota Press. Michael Taussig has given me so much inspiration that it is difficult to isolate a single point or passage of his to cite. His influence is evident in every sentence and idea. Jennifer Wicke meticulously read through chapters time and again, providing invaluable commentary, as did Carolyn Dever. Anne McClintock assisted with brilliant questions, suggestions, and conversations.

I feel lucky to know some remarkably generous people. Kenneth J. Saltman has been an amazing intellectual force, providing me with countless intellectual challenges and clarity, keeping me focused on the important political issues. Many of the most quintessential ideas in this book were thrashed out in conversations with him or by reading books together. He spent an immense amount of time, devotion, and care listening to me read through parts of this text and offering, in response, his ingenious insights. Daniela Peluso read through chapters on numerous occasions and suggested essential recommendations, articles, and encouragement. Michel Alexiades has contributed his excellent scientific credentials and expertise, as well as subscribing me, behind my back, to *Natural History.* Lenio Myrivili and Daniela Gandolfo both moved in with me for weeks at a time, spread drafts out on the floor, and attacked those drafts with hard and helpful critique. Monica Von Thun Calderón provided untold assistance, support, resources, cooking, hospitality, formatting, and printing. To Rona and Allen Goodman, I owe everything.

I consulted many people during the course of preparing this book. Some read and critiqued drafts of chapters; others provided essential materials, advice, or information. I wish to thank all those who contributed their comments, their editing, and/or their logistical support at various stages in the development of this work: Timothy Reiss, Sylvia Molloy, Paul Julian Smith, Lisa Duggan, Dorothy Nilken, Donald Lovett, Martin Van Delden, Margaret Cohen, Barbara Price, Debbie Poole, Avital Ronell, Terrance Turner, Brian Ferguson, Cecilia McCallum, Daryl Posey, Dwight H. Purdy, Diana Robins, Nancy Huse, Milly Seubert of the film department at the Smithsonian's Museum of the American Indian, Geoffrey O'Connor, Mel Lawrence, Kathy McMillan, Drew Walker, Dorothy Chansky, Christopher Davis, Kate Ramses, Heather Simmons, John Stoney, Jim Lahey, Dalia Kandiyoti, Shari Huhndorf, Hannah Feldman, Mandy Harris, Sylvia Vega-Llona, Fabiola Daly, Gracia Aljovín, Alvaro Valarde, Freddy Cooper, Rosario de Bedoya, Maruja Barrig, the members of Flora Tristán, of CENDOC, and of Manuela Ramos. I would also like to thank the Department of Comparative Literature at New York University for funding the research in Peru and for the intellectual rigor they demanded of me while I was studying and writing there, and the Feminist Research Institute of the University of New Mexico for supporting the project in its later stages. I also thank the Graduate Faculty at the New School for Social Research, the Graduate Feminist Forum at New York University, the American Comparative Literature Association, the Feminist Research Institute at the University of New Mexico, and the Women's Center of the College of New Jersey for allowing me to present and discuss sections of this book while in production.

Introduction

> *What would it mean ... to consider the assumption of sexual positions, the disjunctive disordering of the human as "masculine" or "feminine" as taking place not only through a heterosexualizing symbolic with its taboo on homosexuality, but through a complex set of racial injunctions which operate in part through the taboo on miscegenation. Further, how might we understand homosexuality and miscegenation to converge at and as the constitutive outside of a normative heterosexuality that is at once the regulation of a racially pure reproduction.*
>
> —Judith Butler, *Bodies That Matter*

In the nineteenth century, evolutionary sciences brought to the forefront of scientific investigation interspecial crossings as the dominant factor in adaptive biological change. Earlier, following on the work of Linnaeus, species were classified according to their reproductive affinities and whether they could produce fertile offspring. Darwin's observations in the field of domestic breeding reconsidered, as permeable, the reproductive barriers that had previously defined the parameters of species but did not completely do away with them. "We must, therefore," Darwin asserted, "either give up the belief of the universal sterility of the species when crossed; or we must look at this sterility in animals, not as an indelible characteristic, but as one capable of being removed by domestication" (Darwin, 1993: 370). This re-examination of reproductive barriers lent support to one of Darwin's major contributions to the field of biology: that there was no distinction between species and varieties, and new species could therefore emerge from old species' reproducing. Priorly invested with the configurative power of segregating species, infertility became, at the same time, the very gateway to evolutionary transcendence, optimal adaptability, competitive advantage, and perfectibility. The historical placement of absolute unreproductivity on the border of the species concept was, without ever disappearing, transformed, within studies of plant and animal domestication, into a site of uncertain meaning, blurring definitions, and unsettled categories.

Within the stories told to chronicle evolutionary history, female infertility is a central motif that causes a whole host of biological transformations to occur. Female infertility instigates a gap in the trajectory of the evolutionary tale. In this gap the male acquires the adaptable features defining a new special essence. The temporal gap opened by female infertility is an imminent threat of arrest in the evolutionary process—a threat that, at the same time, goads evolution on. In other words, female sexual restraint gives impetus to a male desire for superseding, for mastery. The identity of a species comes to emerge, within the narratives of natural history, as a moment of masculine development brought into play by female reproductive postponements. This figuring of female infertility as the border of evolutionary adaptability and biological change would have repercussions within subsequent understandings of female sexuality, its narratives, social placements, attributions, and the identities formed in its symbolic webs.

As reproduction and female fertility is, ultimately, the unquestioned basis for considering sexual difference and defining genders, infertility can upset the stability of categories based on the phallus, the name and its heredity. Female unreproductiveness codes the suspense in the plotting of Oedipal narratives, where the prohibitive barriers placed on the mother threaten the course of the little boy's development and his ego's survival. Yet also, Oedipal narratives' failures—hysterical symptoms, sexual aberrations, and homosexuality in women—are points of reference to historical periods when the scarcity of resources put limits on reproduction and when libidinal drives had to be redirected, precariously, into the moral and intellectual activities at the base of civilization's development. Colonial encounters were likewise recounted in historical and fictional discourses where morality, constituting the backbone of civilization, was seriously endangered and put into crisis through men's lack of access to European women, the subsequent institutionalization of concubinage, and other sorts of domestic arrangements with women in the colonies.

Interacting with stories of female withdrawals from sex is the Enlightenment ideal of nature's domination by capitalist expansion and the growth of cultures of reason. Max Horkheimer and Theodor Adorno (1991), Frankfurt School critical theorists, argued in their celebrated critique of the Enlightenment that nature was what capitalism aimed to seize and destroy: "Men have always had to choose between their subjection to nature or the subjection of nature to the Self. With the extension of the bourgeois commodity economy, the dark horizon of myth is illumined by the sun of calculating reason, beneath whose cold rays the seed of the new barbarism grows to fruition" (32). Nature resists domination in order to confirm the ultimate power of reason to overcome and possess it. For Horkheimer and Adorno, nature—in the form of myth, magic, and superstition—is being dominated by an emerging fascism that seeks to appropriate nature's powers. As Kate Soper (1996) has suggested, such thinking has led to a positioning of nature as always exterior to social and productive activities, always being acted upon by human endeavor, in the name of progress. Reflecting the basis of environmental preservation, this view constructs an idealized nature that must be "saved" from the discordant and deathly uses to which instrumental rationality has subjected it. "Untamed nature begins to figure as a positive and redemptive power," Soper observes,

> only at the point where human mastery over its forces is extensive enough to be experienced as itself a source of danger and alienation. It is only a culture which has begun to register the negative consequences of its industrial achievements that will be inclined to return to the wilderness, or to aestheticize its terrors as a form of foreboding against further advances upon its territory. (25)

Redeeming a precapitalist moment before industrial technology would control laboring bodies, nature is reconsidered, within natural history, as a romantic and inaccessible object of desire with the potential of eluding the grasp, temporarily, of a dangerously technologized world. The narratives of a nature brought, sometimes brutally, under rational and technological mastery, parallel the tales of natural science—where female sexual resistance constitutes the catalyst of evolutionary progress in masculine development—by situating females as always the exterior, just beyond reach, spurring domination. The domination of nature thesis, retold as a story of scientific knowledge, is violently realized in images of conquest and rape.

Not only in scientific worlds but also in social spheres, unreproductivity was becoming, in the late nineteenth century, an anxious focus demonstrating a crisis at the center of social life. The medical professions' and institutions' growing involvement in the control of female reproduction talks about a general sense of crisis over population rates. Despite the preponderance of evidence purporting women's much earlier involvement in practices like midwifery, contraception, and many forms of abortion in the nineteenth century, women's control over their reproductivity became, as Carroll Smith-Rosenberg and Charles Rosenberg (1973), among others, have remarked, a focus of concern for medicine. As Ornella Moscucci (1990) has shown, this control became the basis for the institutionalization of medical specializations like surgery, general practitioning, and, of course, gynecology. Discourses about contraception, feminism, the education of women, or wartime mortalities arose, in part, from worries about who was reproducing what and where, and how racial lineages could be drawn within a colonial situation that was no longer absolutely authoritative or effectually stable. In fact, a crisis in late-nineteenth century colonial relations can be observed within the articulations of declining birth rates and the regulation of sexualities. Affecting the way female sexualities would be defined, the focus on rates of reproductivity created ambiguities in colonial relations, policy, and controls.

What interests me here is the way colonial relations were and global economies continue to be reschematized as domestic narratives and family stories. As Ann Laura Stoler (1995) has observed, colonial power infiltrated, through housekeeping journals and moral guidelines for educating children, the enclosure of the family, seeking to maintain European identity pure of colonial contagion. However, by anxiously guarding the borders of the home, colonial authority was marking it, its feminine sphere, and the economic system that sustained it, as already racially tainted and endangered. As a result, Stoler elaborates, the home was a site demanding scrutiny and defense from the biological/cultural assault on the moral fiber of European children, their socialization, and the development of their desires and sexualities. Because the divisions and boundaries on which colonial legal authority depended were being drawn within domestic discourses of female sexuality, they were becoming increasingly undetectable, confused, and untenable, hence increasingly and emphatically bolstered.

If one of my intentions here is to talk about the ways domesticity inhabits colonial and postcolonial discourses, another is to analyze how colonial histories, inscribed in narratives of postcolonial identity, construct gender relations. In the literatures and events assessed in this book, the histories of colonialism, their narratives and symbolic possibilities, provide a fantasy of origins—a primal scene of traumatic conception, both cultural and individual—shaped into strategies for imagining identities, conflicts, autonomy, values, nationalisms, resistances, and the like. The writers and filmmakers whom I discuss have found ways of thinking about contemporary operations of power and the new imperialisms; they constitute colonial history as a site of radical rupture and resistance to colonizing power, as much as a point where colonial values and structures of authority can be repeated and reinstituted. The gendering of colonial practices within these texts recreates the painful legacies of empire as romantic tales of affiliative desire and, ultimately, of union, but also as violent historical breaks symbolized in scenes of rape.

In what follows, I read canonical works, locating them within cultural and global movements. Linking the literary analysis to landmark events—a national election in Peru, an earth summit in Brazil—or epistemological settings—the development of a "magic realist" regionalist aesthetic, the medicalization of women's sexuality—I look at these works as sharing in the constructions of historical discourses and contemporary debates over ethnic representation, racial identities, and the politics of reproduction. This book covers a vast amount of ground and a wide array of material. While rooting my readings within social histories and movements, I look at the conjunction between scientific, political, and cultural fields of production, focusing on a variety of types of texts: novels, literary traditions, statements of aesthetic intent, anthropology, journalism, environmentalism, primary biological and psychoanalytic studies, cultural theory, and ethnographic video, among others.

In the first chapter, "Darwin's Dating Game," I discuss the influence of evolutionary theory on Havelock Ellis's and Sigmund Freud's analyses of sexual difference in women. The nineteenth-century biological sciences used sexual difference to mark progress in evolutionary development. For Freud, I argue, the biogenetic law of bisexuality explained periodic returns of the primitive during the female cycle with its privileged relationship to ancestral and racial memories in the unconscious. The logic of recapitulation (individual development literally repeats special development), through which Freud formulates his developmental theories of the psyche, envisions female inaccessibility to male sexual advances as a sign of danger in the evolutionary process as well as in the individual's pathway to civilization and maturity. Meanwhile, Ellis would mark the difference between civilization and savagery by juxtaposing the institution of modesty—the conscious female manipulation instituting civilization's foundational rituals in gender games—to "real" abstinence among animals and savages based on a disinterest due to periodic biological cycles. Such critical, even foundational, models of female sexuality, even as they inform contemporary feminist critiques, embrace Darwin's original configuration of infertility as a biological effect of domestication, hybridization, and female selection.

In the second chapter, "Conrad's Closet," I show another site where femininity is constituted as a racial border by exploring the ways in which racial mixing in the colonies, as treated in Joseph Conrad's earliest novels *Almayer's Folly* and *An Outcast of the Islands*, marks his later representation of the "New Woman" in *Chance*. Centering the symbolic production of motherhood as a defense of colonial authority within Conrad's texts, I argue that Flora's "unnatural" unreproductiveness, and her contingent political subjectivity and self-sufficiency, are heavily reliant on the hidden internal presence of black femininity. I also show that the "unnaturalness" of gender, its artificiality, is deeply connected with the growth of global capital speculation and advertising, giving rise to a new understanding of money circulating as an item of universal exchange outside of any reference or contingency to material value. In this intertextual reading of Conrad, I map, through their gender positions, the ambiguities instituted through colonialism's hybrid identities, situating discourses of female reproductive biologies at the core of postcolonial ambivalences while exploring how such ambivalences are manufactured through networks of global capital.

Then, with the third chapter, "Carpentier's Marvelous Conception," I move into Latin American settings where gender becomes a salient factor in the construction of nationalist narratives. One of the ways, for example, that the Cuban novelist Alejo Carpentier creates "Latin American" literary difference is by contrasting lesbianism, as a sign of European decadence, with infertile hybridity as a sign of Latin America's particularized cultural histories. As a sign of Western decadence, lesbianism carries within itself the idea of the demise of Western culture (the end of its reproduction) as a result of its saturation in technology and media; there, reality has been mystified, atrophied, and dematerialized in empty signs of commercialism, universal repetition, and exchangeability. In contrast, Latin America's cultures of hybridity, originating in colonial violence, are fully resplendent in joy, freedom, and sexuality. Global economies are thereby encoded into female sexualities as female sexualities, in turn, mark the difference between a dead and unreproductive European modernist expression in surrealism and a vitally alive new Latin American aesthetics. In his "real maravilloso," Carpentier literalizes the shock and chance encounters, which defined surrealist practices, within Latin American histories of conquest and rape as well as in the globalization of the media and its relation to marginal cultures. I further discuss in this chapter how postcolonial theory appropriates the discourse of female inaccessibility, as Carpentier articulates it, to re-envision "Latin American difference" as a symbolic of unintelligibility, as a resistance to epistemological mastery.

In "Mario Vargas Llosa and the Rape of Sebastiana," the fourth chapter, I continue the discussion of female inaccessibility as a problem of knowledge, where female intimacies are shrouded in a secrecy linked to the history of rebellion. The hidden space of female erotics gets inscribed, by Peruvian novelist Mario Vargas Llosa's philosophy of eroticism, as the line conjoining civilization and barbarism, both in Vargas Llosa's literary production and presidential campaign. I here argue that he uses Bataille's theory of eroticism—an absolute unreproductivity—in order to tease out a fantasy of colonial history, with its hierarchies of paternalism, as a destructive obstacle to productive neoliberal capitalist relations. I also assert that the rape of Sebastiana, in Vargas Llosa's 1981 novel *The War of the End of the World (La guerra del fin del mundo)* inscribes a narrative of national cohesion, foundational literary culture, and economic liberalization within an aesthetic defining masculine self-generation as artistic creation. In addition, I show how the symbolic inscription of *la mestiza*—a figure, in counterhegemonic minority literatures, of resistance and escape from linguistic entrapment and objectification—can be equally employed as a discourse that ultimately supports Vargas Llosa's political rhetoric of free market capitalism, multinational expansion, and neoliberalism.

My final chapter, "The Rainforest Rape," treats the internationally covered Palinho Paiakan rape case in Brazil. In that country, debates over constitutional definitions of ethnic identity, ecology, and an anthropology of indigenous media production all played a pivotal role in locating race and gender within new constitutional legislation. Sexual narratives work into the power plays between transnational capitalist interests, cultures of consumption, and technological mediations. Thus, I show how projects of "Indianness," ethnic practice, environmental idealism, political factionalism, territorial contestation, and stereotypes of savagery are inscribed through a spectacular story of rape on the frontier.

One of my concerns in this book is to show how gender operates to create "Latin America" as "the real," the unmediated referent, for modernist aesthetics and, subsequently, for postmodernist and postcolonial theories of hybridity, cultural instability, and linguistic indeterminacy within Latin American criticism and aesthetic and cultural commentary. In addition, I demonstrate how the desire for women comes to symbolize the globalization of national economies, capitalist relations, technologies, and culture.

Many studies of this sort, calling themselves "queer" or some such label where systems of referentiality are called into question, use deconstruction to signify, through the linguistic uprooting of identities, the radicalness of the project. The idea of stepping outside the metaphysics of identity, of de-essentializing linguistic and categorical determinations by demonstrating the mobility of signification, has entered into oppositional discourses like postcolonialism as a fashionable way to explore the possibilities of counterhegemonic thought and action. Superficially cited, however, deconstruction seems to be an overly facile way of thinking about colonial identities as figures of resistance. For example, on the origins of postcolonial narratives in colonial travel literature, Simon Gikandi (1996) says, "Creolity ... can be narrativized as contingent and malleable; it is not fixed by the fetishism of blackness and whiteness inscribed in colonialism's racial taxonomy" (127). Such analysis assumes that certain signifiers are automatically floating ones, while other ones are—again automatically—referentially stuck, without passing through the hard linguistic work of grounding and ungrounding that deconstruction theorizes as the foundation of grammatology.[1] Insisting on the malleability and fluidity of identities and subjective positions puts freedom on a papier-mâché pedestal. What such perspectives neglect is that deconstruction, as a source structure, a way of reading for feminism and postcolonialism and a host of other theoretical articulations of oppositionality, posits essentialism and groundedness as the baseline possibility for ungrounding essentialisms. In other words, fixed essences can only be called into doubt and iterability through, paradoxically, their insistent affirmation. Through "play," the centrally operative power through which deconstruction can begin to be thought, deconstruction allows the possibility that floating signification on the one hand, and fetishization on the other, are, essentially speaking,[2] the same thing. Questioning the logic of referentiality and the metaphysics of identity could be a radical insight but one that is not necessarily, or automatically, or always so. More interesting, perhaps, would be thinking about why questioning referentiality—so popular in academic writing these days—functions as an immediate call to liberation, as resistance and opposition, and even redemption, within contemporary, particularly poststructuralist, discourses.

Judith Butler (1997) is, in my evaluation, the critic who has most clearly and carefully articulated the difficulty of using deconstruction as an exemplary overturning of hegemonic power or as a promise of freedom. For her, performativity and its correlative, subjective agency, require the unmitigated repetition of oppressive structures of power in the same gesture as their subversion. In a critique of Foucault, Butler calls this simultaneous repetition and resignification of the law the "non-place of subversion":

> Consider the inversions of "woman" and "woman," depending on the staging and address of their performance, of "queer" and "queer," depending on pathologizing or contestatory modes. Both examples concern, not an opposition between reactionary and progressive usage, but rather a progressive

> usage that requires and repeats the reactionary in order to effect a subversive reterritorialization.... The law turns against itself and spawns versions of itself which oppose and proliferate its animating purposes. (99–100)

What is clear is that for Butler, one cannot simply reject an ontological investment by crumpling it up and throwing it away or by singularly declaring it null and void. What is clear as well is that the field of sexuality for Butler is a particularly difficult site for analyzing power as resistance, because sexuality itself has particularly strong ties to the hegemonic power of the state and its disciplinary apparatuses: "Disciplinary apparatus fails to repress sexuality precisely because the apparatus is itself eroticized, becoming the occasion for the *incitement of sexuality* and, therefore, undoing its own repressive aims" (101). She does not, however, take it further, in this context, to explore how the sexualization of disciplinary power and the eroticization of the law function inside representations of colonial authority as a locus where desire gets produced and where identities are performed. This is not her failing but rather a challenge to those who question the formulaic appropriation of linguistic indeterminacy as a radical break from power in colonial discourses and postcolonial theories.

Deconstruction and its adherents do offer philosophical insights into the ways identities of self and other are experienced as shaped through an inescapable interaction between metaphysics and dialectical thought. Yet, they do not, for the most part, succeed in showing how such a philosophical perspective interfaces with a world steeped in injustice or with a politics of engagement. It is, admittedly, very important to realize that an oppositional gesture's meaning is likely to be reappropriated or subject to flux, and that the hard foundations of identities are tough to think oneself out of; yet subversions are still possible. In Butler, what results is a confusion of allegiances at the level of subjectivity, where it seems that the critic is so invested in the text and the implementation of the law as to be unable to sustain an oppositional stand. "The subject's existence," she claims in her most recent work on Althusser's theory of interpellation, "cannot be linguistically guaranteed without passionate attachment to the law. This complicity at once conditions and limits the viability of a critical interrogation of the law. One cannot criticize too far the terms by which one's existence is secured" (129). The question remains: Why not? What are the terms of existence that need so much protection, for whom are they secure, and who, in the end, gets the best of them?

What is, therefore, disturbing in Butler's work is the central role that ambiguity plays in tracing political projects or agendas for social change. For Butler, every action that opposes power feeds it at the same time. The position that every act of resistance is also imprecated in power follows from a reworking of a Foucauldian paradigm where power itself produces subjects; subjects in turn are granted political agency and even, at certain historical moments, produce calls for reform, resistance, or revolution. But Butler further contends that "hegemony also works through and as its 'resistance' so that the relation between the marginalized community and the dominative is not, strictly speaking, oppositional" (139). Still, it is usually not very difficult to discern where power imbalances and injustices prevail, who benefits, whose well-being the future of power serves, and who gets trammeled in the process.

In the case of *Paris Is Burning,* for example, Butler argues that the desire of black and Hispanic ball-dancers to identify with white femininity both repeats heterosexual norms and subverts them, demonstrating the artificiality of family, kinship, and heterosexuality by showing their naturalness as performed, that is, as always being constituted and reconstituted. It is not difficult, however, to read where power operates to maintain racial hierarchies in support of keeping economic marginals in a position of desperation. In *Paris Is Burning,* transsexual reorderings of gender necessitate the acquisition of consumer goods through which masculinity, femininity, and whiteness are articulated. Even, as Butler says, the character Venus Xtravaganza's wish "to find a man and have a house in the suburbs with a washing machine" clearly does not challenge in any way the power of white heterosexual codifications. Her corpse, found three days dead under the bed in a sleazy hotel room, surely testifies "that there are cruel and fatal social constraints" (1993: 133) involved in exposing the lie. Though Butler is able to explore how the camera grants the possibility of alternative and even counterhegemonic identities in its production of new desires, the prevalent desire for whiteness and the incessant, unwavering impetus to consume its products and apparel—to spend more than one has in order to become what one can never be—certainly imply that identities are constituted in relation to capital and markets, and that identities formed through control of economic viability are the ones everyone wants to assume but can only assume in play. In the world if not in the text, agency, blame, and human suffering are equally decidable, equally legible. It is usually very clear, even glaring, against whom or what to direct an oppositional critique. One might then ask, Who is it that cannot decide the undecidable, and whose interests are being articulated in the recourse to interpretive ambiguity to which deconstructive readings are prone?

Infertilities does the important work of showing how femininity is integral to thinking about the postcolonial. The globalization of capitalism was and still is forcing change in ideas about gender and its relation to the growth of capital and markets. Such change may spur challenges to current market configurations: today, women comprise 70 percent of the global population that is below the poverty line, and poorly paid and exploited women comprise 70 percent of the workforce in nonindustrialized nations. However, further work needs to be done. *Infertilities* reads through a series of representations and analyzes how the market and capitalism itself have been constructed through the entrenched ideologies of gender, and how gender in turn shapes popular conceptions about markets. Knowing how ideology works is the first step toward suggesting alternatives. It is my hope that such readings help to inspire ideas for social transformation and new possibilities for the future.

Darwin's Dating Game

Mankind dwell in her and she in them. With all men she plays a game for love, and rejoices the more they win. With many, her moves are so hidden, that the game is over before they know it.

—"Nature: Aphorisms by Goethe," *Nature* (4 November 1869)

In its 8 March 1997 issue, *Science* published an article by Julien Thomas entitled "The Mystery of the Missing Penis." In it, Thomas describes a recent biological discovery: certain species of birds, through evolutionary processes, have lost their penises. The reason for this anatomical distinction in birds is, he concludes, "because females prefer them without it." According to Thomas's surprisingly literal citation of a long-since refuted sociobiological model, such a female bird, "in order to maximize her reproductive fitness ... wants to choose the best sperm.... Females have most control over males without an organ. So, the researchers reason, they could be chosen more frequently and would eventually have had greater success than those who wasted their sperm." The result is that such birds reproduce through a "cloacal kiss."

"The mystery ..." repeats a frequently told evolutionary tale where adaptation is measured as an acquisition of masculine traits determined through female choice. Threats to evolutionary masculinity are figured as the result of both environmental hazards and female sexual scarcity. "Like knights from the Arthurian legend," begins, for example, Simon Pollard in *Natural History*, "two male jumping spiders maneuvering for battle unsheathe a pair of long swords and approach each other with fixed stares. The brief clash, which involves much pushing and shoving, is a contest of strength, most likely to gain a chance to mate with any nearby females"

(44). If reproduction is the aim and the end of competition and adaptive survival necessary for evolution to occur, female sexual restraint from males is designated as both the obstacle in which evolution gets suspended and the proof that these males, and their genes, are, indeed, selected as superior, more valuable. Masculinity encoded as both strength and violence represents a special adaptability in strategies of reproduction as narrative[1] foreplay for evolutionary success, an adaptability that would then be transmitted to the next generation of male offspring. In the same issue of *Natural History*, Paul Watson's article, "Dancing in the Dome: Males Are Lured by Food and Sex into Erotic Contests and Deadly Brawls," has a caption that reads, "Two males, with their pedipalps extended, square off to do battle for an egg-laden female. Sexually mature females that remain unmated for a [*sic*] least a week will soak the web with a male-attracting chemical" (43). In the time always preceding the propagation of genetic material, these spiders engage in a process of seduction, with the male embodying the anatomical features necessary for the hunt, and the female endowed with the physical features and entrapment mechanisms beneficial for being pursued as well as a rational agenda for deciding what would make her better off. Warlike competition between males produces a suspenseful tale where the strong and courageous, by winning the promise of fertilization, are granted greater and more numerous futures. "A carnivore that silently stalks and feeds on other slugs, the 'sea tiger' will even attack members of its own species," reads a caption by Richard Milner in another issue of *Natural History.* "Both blind and deaf, it must follow a chemical trail exuded by its prey. Then, using its large, hooklike toothed redula to pull its victims into its mouth, the foot-long predator swallows them whole." In the worlds of popular natural history, females await while the sperm contend for position, fighting off, killing, or, in this case, eating other males in order to win the prize of fertilization. Males enter into violent contests with one another in order to survive through genetic transmissions. Competitive strategies and anatomical advantages are presented as evolving within the gaps of a reproductive outcome that is always awaiting conclusion.

A question that needs to be asked is why evolution has become such a widespread concern in public discussion, from movies such as *Jurassic Park* to *Time* magazine editorials and curricular debates. Evolution foregrounds a language of competition that feeds a triumphant sentiment about the market, ordaining it with nature's grace and upholding it as the only possible way of life. In the evolutionary scenes such as those I described above, it is clear that economic models underpin the gendering of struggle. The feature elements within these developmental trajectories in biology—notions such as competition, value, efficiency, and shortage, which set the parameters for economic rationalism and capitalist expansion—naturalize inequality and unfairness in economic relations. Economic gains and mastery result from psychological desires, isolated choices, and individual passions on the margins, rather than from systemic oppressions like the opposition of interests between labor and capital. Domination rises from an individual's calculation of pleasure and pain—probability and chance—rather than from institutional advantage. That corporate and media interests are involved in the policing of evolutionary stories is evident in, say, the corporate sponsorship of museum exhibits. Universal Pictures, the producers of Steven Spielberg's *The Lost World: Jurassic Park*, for example, supported "The Lost World: The Life and Death of Dinosaurs" at the Museum of Natural History in New York (see Silverstein). What needs to be foregrounded is that evolutionary narratives are actually complicit in producing discourses of corporate culture and consumerism through, among other things, their language of competition, struggle, aesthetic spectacle, acquisition, scarcity, and, in particular, choice. Furthermore, evolutionary thought subjects such insinuations of corporate controls through tales of seduction that naturalize the material history of capital and power.

Evolution is a gradual, heritable change in a population over time. It operates predominantly through natural selection, which is not a force but a process, a result, a random change in the frequency of alleles in a population. Natural selection is noncognitive, so the emphasis, in some of these reproductive battle scenes and romantic interludes, on rational choice and desire, serves to psychologize and individuate—and capture in a photographic moment—a gradual historical change happening to a group in a particular environmental niche; therefore, its ideological basis needs to be investigated, its assumptions unpacked. Basically, Darwin opened the question of how the mixing of forms in reproduction could lead to the emergence of new forms rather than returning to the medium norm of a population. He contributed the theory of natural selection as the strong mechanism that would explain such special transformations. However, Darwin did not solve the problem of evolution because his theory could not adequately explain transmission. It was not until 1900, when Mendel's theories on genetics were "rediscovered," and then in the 1930s, with the modern synthesis explaining natural selection as operating through genetics, that neo-Darwinism, asserting a mixture of inheritance and environmental influence, was ushered in with the theoretical force and nearly universal acceptance it has today. What is at stake in perpetuating such romantic narratives as the modus operandi of change? Containing choice within an individual life story of a quest for individual survival, the evolutionary imperative to reproduce—quickly and abundantly in the face of environmental threats and female inaccessibility—not only precludes the possibility of the collective but also catapults images of eventual familial happiness and splendor as the natural rationale for capitalist accumulation, appropriation, the expansion of the resource base, and an ideology of justice embedded in the maintenance of class privilege.

Though recent research has analyzed the gendering of the evolutionary story, the ways such a gendering feeds ideologies of economic oppression has not aroused so much attention. In the 1970s, Sally Slocum speculated on the origins of human culture and ingenuity in cooperation, childrearing and food gathering rather than in aggression and the production of weapons. Following on Slocum's work, Linda Marie Fedigan, for example, has traced the history of evolutionary thought from a story about "man the hunter" to a much more flexible paradigm, influenced by feminist criticism and supported by ethnographic observations, where gathering is the dominant subsistence activity. Fedigan writes, "Thus, a picture of women as active, competent, contributing, and even self-sufficient members of hunter-gatherer societies, with their own stories to tell, has begun to emerge from the shadows of early ethnographic scenarios" (46). The point seems to be a "let me in" "me-too"-ism, where scientific accuracy would be sharpened through allowing women into management positions, credit opportunities, grant considerations, and other sorts of middle-class living arrangements and institutions of efficiency. A call for equality of access to the cultural sites where inequality is practiced seems to coat such valuations of competence and efficiency as the main agendas for feminism. States

Adrienne Zhilman, "Whether or not there is a conscious effort to keep women in their place, these pervasive attitudes impose a 'glass ceiling' on our female ancestors, much like the 'glass ceiling' that limits the upward occupational mobility of contemporary women both within and outside of the academic disciplines" (1997: 91). This is tantamount to saying that everything would be better if only women, too, were allowed to become nuclear engineers and build bombs. As new speculations about evolution reinterpret the meaning of the available evidence, the struggle between the genders—which evolution still retains as its fundamental code—seems to obscure the class positions that fire the struggle. It is not a broader inclusion into the economy that is needed for fairness but an altogether different vision for the evolutionary future.

The feminist critique of evolution is calling for a broader inclusiveness in science, but this inclusiveness seems to be defined as middle-class mobility. Defining motherhood as a practice of financial hard-dealing, Adrienne Zihlman has argued that females were more active in evolution than the standard Darwinian model would warrant. Reproduction, caring, and nurturing, Zihlman contends, "marked female investment of time and energy in gestating, lactating, and caring for offspring" (1995: 432). In the seventies, Nancy Tanner and Adrienne Zihlman published an influential two-part study in *Signs,* which argued that females did play a part in evolutionary progress through their role as nurturers and socializers, protecting gene life and controlling transmissions: "Influencing the evolutionary direction of the species, they invested time and energy in their offsprings' survival (maternal investment) and chose as their mates those males more protective and willing to share food than the average male ape (sexual selection)" (1978: 4). Females actively select the genes they want their kids to have by waiting to see which males will be the bigger and better providers, the ones more skilled at acquisitions. Females withdraw their reproductive labor until they can be assured the evolutionary profit. Models of evolution that include females as agents seem simply to extend, even to motherhood, the economic rationalism of investment as an ever-deeper lure, the fantasy of a broader-based consumption.

The economics of evolution have, always, indeed produced female agents. Darwin himself determined the value of trait acquisitions through female sexual selection. The idea of choice—of natural environmental selection and, later, female choice—marks evolutionary theories about gender as tied to an emergent consumerist ideal of commodity variability. Margaret Schabas has argued that Victorian biology avoided considerations of political economy. Nineteenth-century economic science understood the social as a field of rational agency veering away from the natural. The focus on psychology as the ground for the development of species actually opposed contemporary nineteenth-century political economic adherents such as David Ricardo. Instead, evolution demonstrated a web of intersecting deliberations always tending naturally toward the common good, as in the older liberal theories of political economy proposed by Adam Smith and others. Though Schabas does expose interesting contradictions between nineteenth-century developments of evolutionary biology and political economy, she nevertheless neglects to see the autonomy of the mind in psychology as precisely contingent on specific economic forces. Psychology arises in the nineteenth century alongside, say, a growth in international trade, an increasing rationalization of labor in manufacturing, and the resultant alienation of workers. It also hinges on the expansion of the market, the proliferation of an increasingly varied selection of goods, the speeding up of the new and the innovative in available technologies and products, and a concomitant outgrowth of a consumer culture based on an ideology of individual choice. Critics of science, such as Ruth Hubbard and Cynthia Eagle Russet, have noted how configurations of power emerging out of industrialization, divisions of labor, and the growing internationalization of capital informed the ways power was imagined within evolutionary science.[2] Hubbard, for example, concludes that "Darwin's interpretation of the history of life on earth not only fits well into the social doctrines of nineteenth-century liberalism and individualism but was used, in turn, to support them by rendering them aspects of natural law" (92). Even if Victorian science was not in line with contemporaneous theories of the economy, it certainly did—and does still—express an understanding of the economy as operating under the laws of nature. This naturalization of economic injustices, in turn, produced gender as already implicating hierarchies and power struggles.

The idea that scarcity results from individual psychology, decision making, or the personal tastes of finicky females, positions scarcity as independent of the economy and, more than that, beyond anybody's blame. "For our purposes, male-male competition can be defined as competition for female gametes and the resources a female might allocate to them" (Barrett and Warner, 335). The idea that females control the allocation of resources feeds current policy debates over welfare, for example, allocating blame for unjust resource distribution to its very victims. The prevailing evolutionary metaphor exhibiting male competition for access to females repeats a Malthusian model based on scarcity. Andrew Ross has noted how ecological thought, governed by "the law of competition" and "the condition of scarcity" (106), is conceived in line with a culture of consumption that perceives abundance on the wane and earlier excesses providing a margin of economic sin.[3] Within such thought, females are constituted as the reason for scarcity. Heterosexual desire is the only promise of overcoming an originary, inevitable lack; reproduction is the only path toward economic solvency. There is no sense here of a general economy that actually depends on distributions of scarcity in order to create wealthy little enclaves, speedy production, a surplus of labor, and ever-narrower zones of accumulation; no sense of what kinds of agents benefit from such a set-up. The centrality of scarcity in the labor of evolution implies that underproduction and natural deficiencies pose challenges to survival and even extinction, whereas individual effort, displays of strength, and forbearance can overcome the challenge. The same metaphor says that nature is a place of constant consumption, where the largest consumers prevail. What such a model assumes is the ultimate usefulness of all activity and the rationality behind all organic form and all development. It belies the changes that occur through the overabundance of production, the plenitude of nature, and the control over consumption exerted not by the frugalities of nature but by those who command the forces of production and have monopolies over the technologies of desire.

Assuming nature as always invested in a play of provisional limits, evolution shows the acquisition of wealth as the organic growth of bodily strength and the persistence, indeed the overproduction of a healthy, protective, instinctual, individualized desire. In other words, evolution envisions a debt structure as already part of nature. Just as with the Christian law of paying-back in guilt and devotion for salvation, debt and lack are figured as female sexuality that, holding back on provisions, insatiably insists on expenditure, sacrifice, and investment for transcendent survival: "The conviction reigns that it is only through the sacrifices and accomplishments of the ancestors that the tribe *exists*—and that one has to *pay them back* with sacrifices and accomplishments: one thus recognizes a *debt* that constantly grows greater" (Nietzsche, 88–89). Within public debates over the place of evolution in curricula, the seemingly raging and enduring conflict between evolutionism and creationism—where it is important, indeed absolutely vital and necessary, that evolutionism ends up universally adopted—tends to obscure the gender politics, feminine subordination, and class struggle in which both evolutionism and creationism similarly concur. Evolution participates in, indeed creates, a culture of endless and relentless consumption.

Gender provides a door through which class divisions can operate as natural catalysts to evolution. Gender and reproduction give rise to the struggle for power. Evolution has posited the origin of species within romantic narratives of sex, where the courtship is won through the acquisition of more robust and competitive features of maleness. The more attractive traits would be chosen by the mate because they would ensure to a greater degree her own chances for survival. See, for example, Carl N. Degler's discussion of turn-of-the-century feminist sociology, especially his treatment of Lester Frank Ward's *Pure Sociology* (1903): "Thus she chooses the mate who is stronger and bigger than the others, as well as those with moral attributes like courage and beauty" (1991: 111). Sex difference encoded the evolutionary tale by ushering in a romantic schematization—the delays, mysteries, and overcoming of obstacles, the hunt for the means to propagate and therefore survive—in the pursuit of evolutionary advantage. As Ruth Bernard Yeazell has observed, "For Darwin . . . , to study sex is to find already inscribed in Nature a familiar narrative of courtship—a narrative about female resistance . . . that English middle-class culture had been telling itself for more than two hundred years" (34). Evolution sets power in place through sex, constituting gender itself inside of an initial battle for resources in a war over production and consumption. Such narrative images of evolution have been remarkably uniform and persistent since the Victorian era. One might argue that they are historically contingent and demand that at different moments such stories take on different forms. The tenacity of this evolutionary romance—female restraint and individualized choice; male competition, supersedence, and final acquisition—however, testifies that underlying it is an intensely dominant and even unshakable program that has defined social practices since the mid-nineteenth century, a cultural imaginary based in a logic of consumption.

In evolution, female sexuality functions as a limit to exactly what masculinity can do and acquire—a limit to growth, a limit to population[4] and the value that accrues to it, a limit to wealth and the struggle to attain it. Yet, female sexuality also makes masculinity productive, causing it to perform ever more elaborate tasks to please it, or to create ever more beautiful traits to attract it. Evolution relies on attributing roles to gender that justify capital. In an environment whose provisions are constantly depleting, the male's victory, in the quest for food and survival, figures as his struggle, against all odds, to overcome and control female reproductive scarcity. In the face of female restraint, males must develop, the logic goes, the necessary equipment, cunning, and superior abilities to lure the female into reproduction, by nurturing her and protecting her, and to fight off those who might arrive there first. This assumes the female separately constituted outside of economic activity and competition, where the care and socialization of the young is removed from the fight for dominance and ascendance in which males exclusively engage. Female restraint operates as a narrative through which resource depletion is inserted into the evolutionary tale; some win access to the remaining scarce resources while others die. Femininity here professes that economic scarcity is a natural feature of biological development, and that class struggle may be about physical stamina, masculine ingenuity, and feminine coyness rather than about a playing field that always favors some over others because of race, class, gender, national citizenship, institutional affiliation, family name, capital acquisition, financial backing, legalized inequities, media control, corporate consolidation, political clout, prejudice, or ultimate primacy over the means of production.

The critique of science has often failed to take into account the class struggle embedded in the gendering of evolution. Those rethinking objectivity and/or considering how science creates exclusions seem often to be making a liberal call for extending the parameters of inclusion, insinuating that assimilation would lead to fairness, rather than proposing to restructure the terms, affiliations, paradigms, and institutions through which science asks its questions and tells its stories. For example, Sandra Harding suggests, "When women or men scientists can figure out how to ask questions about nature's regularities . . . , the storehouse of human scientific knowledge can expand and the knowledge will become more accurate" (199). All we need to do, says Harding, is expand knowledge, let it extend into places never before explored, in the name of Truth with a capital "T." This type of "solution" to problems posed by objectivity posits that more knowledge can only be better for everybody, assuming that more of a variety of middle-class people embraced by more middle-class institutions can bring about social change or, at the very least, change in institutional practices and ways of knowing. Such a recommendation, however, does not adequately challenge the historical propensity of science to oppress people *precisely through inclusion.* The Hegelian dialectic pictures a science-subject that assimilates the unknown through force and violence, turning the object ever more thoroughly into itself. Likewise, the Human Genome Project extends its collecting ever more deeply into the Fourth World, cataloguing blood types from people who have never before seen a syringe, just in order to store the samples in laboratories, for the sake of accumulating more knowledge, to the possible benefit of no one except, possibly, multinational pharmaceutical companies. Questions arise: Is more knowledge always good knowledge? Is it sometimes more ethical not to know? In whose interest is the growth of knowledge, and to whom does it give power? As Harding's model for change adds on to the center—through synthesis—an ever-growing number of identities on the margins (what she calls "strong objectivity"), one might seriously ask if what this is all about is that, as Susan Sperling remarks, "now everyone gets to eat power lunches on the savannah" (218). Putting women on the face of science seems to be as promising as putting a female face on, say, the British head of state and expecting things to change for the better. What mere inclusion forgets is that such a project needs to take into account economic redistribution if equality is ever to be achieved.

Harding's idea that gender inclusion would challenge objectivity works to conceal the class exclusion that is operating inside of her model and the conservative liberalism that underlies her agenda for a new science.

Donna Haraway, in contrast, does consider class struggle as a vital factor in understanding the ways science produces genders. For her, the study of biology in particular focuses on the body as the site of various types of oppressions and dominations that become naturalized, expressing ideas of the body politic as, instead, facts about the nature of the body: "Neither our personal bodies nor our social bodies may be seen as natural, in the sense of existing outside of the self-creating process called human labour. What we experience and theorize as nature and as culture are transformed by our work" (10). One may wonder, perhaps, if labor is the only force constructing the identities of our bodies. As it focuses predominantly on the body of the producer—on labor—Haraway's analysis sidesteps the necessarily contingent analysis of how the body itself is implicated in the vast and ever-growing culture of the consumer. Evolutionary paradigms depend on female choice as the cause for various spectacular male flourishes and exhibitions. Evolution is thus expressing, in the struggle between the genders, a type of selection that increasingly craves, even demands, variety, innovation, and spectacle. Female choice, rather than being liberatory, is the naturalization, in the body, of the will to buy.

Built up in cycles of hunger and want, gender functions as a mechanism of repression precisely because it is constituted through shortage. Desire is never fulfilled because there is never enough to go around, and so one must come up with all sorts of wily tricks in order to get enough, to beat the system. Mainstream understandings of reproduction, indeed, pose female reproduction as a limit to available resources where, as Foucault says, "power is situated and exercised at the level of life" (137). In the evolutionary story of competition, female anatomy is depicted as the environmental hazard that endangers the lives of all but the strongest and the cleverest sperm, restricting successful consumption, narrowing access. Judith Roof analyzes such "sperm tales" as presented in the 1980s *Nova* series *The Miracle of Life:*

> The sperm encounter the "dangerously inhospitable" environment of the female vagina where one fourth of the sperm force dies immediately. A large contingent of defective sperm malfunctions. Foreign cells in the woman's body, some healthy sperm are attacked by antibodies. Other deeply anxious sperm hit prematurely on incorrect cells. The remainder swims mightily against contrary currents. (1996: 4)

Male survival is at stake, but the ones who do survive are robust, hearty, and thriving, having proven their potency. Reproduction plays into a grand and uplifting allegory of evolutionary competence. Female sexual disinterest (in heterosexuality), meanwhile, is a mechanism of death, firmly grounded, so to speak, in scare stories about environmental destruction where this disinterest is as fatal as the ruinous toxins invading the air. "In the early Seventies," notes, for example, Jay Rayner in Virgin Atlantic Airline's magazine *Hot Air,*

> Californian researchers noted that female gulls were nesting together—a pattern they soon realized was repeated all over the US. The males appeared to have lost interest. A study of male gulls revealed that they had developed female organs. While the females were turning into lesbians, the males were turning into females.... A few years later scientists studying alligators in Florida discovered an increasing number of males to be rather less endowed than might be expected. More than half of them had tiny penises—fascinating for the scientists and deeply depressing for the alligators. (15)

Such suspension of the developmental narratives of masculinity are caused by the ecological perils of an increasingly technological and commercial modern world. Chemicals released into the air by new industries, or natural contaminants such as female urine in the rivers, "mimic oestrogen" (16), dramatically infecting male fetuses and affecting their sperm counts and fertility successes in adult life.[5] With gulls and alligators sprouting up everywhere as lesbians, female sexuality operates to decrease viable natural resources, as scarcity. Females are at fault for the fatalities caused by pollution and environmental contaminants, rather than industry and corporations.

The figuration of resource scarcity as reproductive scarcity extends, as well, to the processes of human evolution as they are covered in the mainstream media. Often, the environment is imagined as mean, treacherous, and ungiving, and this translates into nonreproductive sexuality. On 25 October 1992, for example, *Time* published a report on the excavation of the Iceman. A 5,300-year-old skeleton, the Iceman was discovered by hikers in the Tyrolean Alps in 1991. His body, which was buried under glacial frost, had quickly mummified, and thus scientists were expecting his remains to reveal truths about how people lived during the Stone Age. The *Time* article also mentions that when the Iceman was recovered, his penis was missing. Nevertheless, the article claims, "several women . . . have volunteered to be impregnated with his sperm" (66) because they do not know what he cannot do. The absurdity of the situation is in the irony of women who, choosing to have something which is so unchoosable and unattractive, will eventually have to come to their senses. The *Time* article repeatedly mentions the women's interest in "having his baby" (62) while, at the same time, constantly emphasizing, through invoking the missing organ, the Iceman's competitive inferiority in the reproductive game, the impossibility of such a consummation symbolized in the missing organ. The illustration of the Iceman accompanying the article depicts him as short, straggly, and thin, bent over with a slightly fearful demeanor and in a defensive pose, a narrow spear suspended in his tightly clenched fist. The Iceman, it is said, went down fighting, being "snatched from life completely outfitted with the implements of everyday existence!" exclaims Markus Egg, the German archaeologist who is overseeing the delicate process of restoring the Iceman's belongings" (62). Stricken down during a hunt for food directly preceding glacial frosts, the Iceman seemed to have been engaged in a struggle for survival against environmental pressures and competition, for access to meager resources for growth and generation, a struggle that he did not have the tools or abilities to win.

Ironically, in 1997, the Iceman comes back as the strong and courageous tamer of the wild, master of his surroundings. As featured in Macmillan/McGraw-Hill's award-winning sixth-grade multicultural social studies textbook *World*, the Iceman, "equipped for survival," represents an original test-case scenario of regional and cultural diversity. Though no mention is made of the Iceman's tragic castration (or of the renowned and slightly frustrated archaeologist, Egg), the tale of his life as survivor has been pieced together by archaeologists through a step-by-step process-analysis of the materials found with him. The illustration of the Iceman shows him now as robust, aggressive, and forward-leaning, as though set for tracking. He has a wide chest, an expression of resolve, a thick and sturdy bow, and a flint knife (termed "survival equipment" in a caption [35]) hanging from his waist, down between his legs. Five years after the initial discovery, the Iceman has come to embody the protomasculine codes of individual fortitude, prowess, and physical stamina, the same qualities missing from his tale of precarious survival and impotency in 1992. His masculinity is emphatically restored as he becomes a hero of survival in a dangerous environment, of hunting skill and intelligent tool-making, of struggle against resource depletion, at the origin of a new human history. There is no longer any talk of the impossibility of women selecting him for propagation, nor the ironic delays caused by his evolutionary lacks and inadequacies, obstacles to his selectability. Presented as possessing the full array of cultural products and outfitted with the instruments of competitive advantage, the Iceman has become father to us all.

These stories, of course, are not new. In 1970s popular scientific literature, for instance, biological paradigms mobilized such images of competition between males over scarce females, with its implied sexual pursuits. Indeed, the interest in sociobiology in the seventies emerges in conjunction with a changing politics of gender and class resulting from the rise of second-wave feminism, price inflation, a cultural terror over what was seen as a global depletion of energy resources, and the idea of the Third World—in the media's vision of OPEC—as a frightening and malignant competitor. Yet, sociobiology itself does not acknowledge the influences of such factors as the new configuration of global trade, the break-up of monopolies, economic tightening, hype over inflation, the intensification of consumerism in the proliferated construction of new shopping centers and malls, or the new freedoms women found in the *Roe v. Wade* Supreme Court decision; instead, sociobiology regulates all struggle for survival to stories of romance, seduction, and male-controlled competition for reproductive fulfillment and clear hereditary lineages. Richard Dawkins's sociobiological game theory envisions a gene with an obsessive agenda for self-propagation. The gene in this theory considers all possibilities in a cost-benefits analysis in order to arrive at the most efficient methods for producing the largest number of offspring with the most minimal amount of energy expenditure. In this assembly-line model for human reproduction, the reward is greater for males since they can reproduce more with less time investment:

> Since a female produces a limited number of eggs at a relatively slow rate, she has little to gain from having a large number of copulations with different males. A male on the other hand, who can produce millions of sperms every day, has everything to gain from as many promiscuous matings as he can snatch. Excess copulations may not actually cost a female much, other than a little lost time and energy, but they do not do her positive good. A

> male on the other hand can never get enough copulations with as many different females as possible. (164)

Evolution, now a suspension between an initial investment and an eventual return, is a story about how tightfisted females with limited funds save and carefully invest their reproductive worth while males are reckless spendthrifts because they naturally have more to squander. Because males are always richer than females in terms of potential quantities of reproduction, the evolutionary imperative to heterosexual union is constituted as managerial excellence, the obvious advantage that males have in business bureaucracies, financial firms, global competition, agencies of speculation, and the growing service economy. Male evolution prepares us for Reagan.

Centralizing reproduction—the economic rationalism pervading sociobiology—is fundamental to evolutionary thought historically. Evolutionary pathways are carved through scenarios of female sexual denial, which naturally institutes a material economic lack. Reproduction since Darwin has been the dominant mechanism through which evolution occurs. Biological science has universally assumed that what distinguishes the human from other species is that in humans, estrus (the phase in the menstrual cycle when the female is fertile) is not seasonal. Evolution has centered this fact as the cause of human social organization; the sexual availability and pleasure of females at all times has tended to explain, for instance, the nuclear family as natural because it increases the reproductive success of both parties as they cooperate in bringing up offspring. Recent feminist scholarship in biology has, however, been able to drive a (heretofore seemingly unmovable) wedge between female sexuality and reproduction. Elisabeth Lloyd, for example, has argued that sexual activities of female animals outside of estrus are generally not observed or remarked by researchers even though they might not be so rare. Yet, female sexual denial continues to indicate a limitation in the availability of natural resources that justifies the ascendance of some over others in the struggle for power. Males must possess either the strength and courage, or the intelligence and skills necessary to prevail in a world where females are constantly limiting their sexual accessibility, demanding to be fed and choosing to be pleased.

Human males therefore develop a wide range of intellectual abilities that set them above the other species just in their capacity to outsmart them, win mates, and pass down genes. Susan Sleeth Mosedale says of Darwinian theory, "Their success is attributed to their ability to overpower or outmaneuver other males in competition over females" (6); therefore, "the greater the 'development' of the race, the greater the difference in skull capacities between male and female" (8). Sexual difference in intelligence signifies a measure of evolutionary progress. Darwin's student George Romanes, for instance, contended that "the marked inferiority of intellectual power" in women, supported in the anatomical evidence of lesser cranial capacities and lesser cranial weights measured against those of men, "is proportionally a greater difference than that between the male and female organisms as a whole, and the amount of it is largely affected by grade of civilization—being least in savages and most in ourselves" (11).

The persistence of competition as a central conceptual metaphor within Darwin's own thought, as well as in that of his contemporaries, foregrounds the importance of competition in defining a world view newly caught in mechanisms of globalization. In addition to the growth of industrialization and the rise of labor movements, the 1857 mutiny against the British colony in India was certainly a factor in challenging Britain's supremacy in the world. Before then, it was believable to think of Britain as governing those who needed to be governed—"savages" and the like. Afterward, the fabric of the empire started to unravel as it was no longer so clear, within metropolitan discourse, that the colonizers were doing good and moral works for people who just needed a little uplifting. Darwin was developing evolutionary thought when the British conception of their role as colonizers was changing. There was a new sense that the colonized would not just be the submissive receivers of British benevolence but would now challenge rule and law, compete for power, make demands for justice, and demonstrate the actual weakness of Britain's hold on imperial power.

It is clear, too, that the central role competition plays in evolutionary thought responds to the undermining of ideas about male superiority waged by the first wave of the feminist movement with its demands for equal education, equal rights to own and inherit property, and, finally, equal participation in politics. Most evolved males who won the competition were, obviously, more intelligent, but greater intelligence would also mark a greater difficulty in reproduction and a greater effort to overcome that difficulty. In an 1875 study, Joseph Taber Johnson, lecturer in obstetrics at Georgetown, for example, argued that the larger cranial sizes of white male babies required conforming changes in pelvis size and shape in white females in comparison to black females, leading, in turn, to more precarious and painful childbirth and longer labors in the "more civilized" races. Robert Morris, a New York doctor, on the other hand, observes that the increasing impressionability of women's nervous systems has led to a degenerative clitoris, with a resulting decrease in sexual desire as civilization advances. The outcome will be, says Morris, that women will do selective breeding, holding out for greater intelligence rather than basing their choices on emotion alone, with contingent downward effects on birth rates. These medical studies relegate women solely to a reproductive role that, as a barrier to male procreation, proves reproductive difficulties are contingent to the increased intelligence of evolved men and, defensively, to the competitive advantage of such intelligence among "the civilized."

What makes "population" such a difficult and salient topic within evolutionary thought is that as much of numerical proliferation was important and, indeed, essential for species' survival, so it overstrained the economic volatility of a particular niche and so caused death—perhaps to entire populations—out of selection. In other words, as species thrived by reproducing a lot, they also threatened themselves with shortages and overcrowding. At the time, there was a widespread social concern over "population" that blamed women and even feminism for a supposedly cataclysmal decline in fertility rates.[6] In W. L. Atlee and D. A. O'Donnell's 1871 report on abortion, the patient of surgical abortion, they say, like the feminist who shirks her social role, "becomes unmindful of the course marked out for her by Providence, she overlooks the duties imposed on her by the marriage contract. She yields to the pleasures—but shrinks from the pains and responsibilities of maternity" and, in the end, is punished with "stains of blood on her soul" (as cited in Smith-Rosenberg and Rosenberg: 350). Referring to feminism, Havelock Ellis himself, in 1892, agreed that "as a general rule the woman who refuses motherhood in order to serve humanity is like a soldier who prepares himself on the eve of battle for the forthcoming struggle by opening his veins" (Weeks: 174). In opposition, some feminists claimed that birth control would save the world from being run over by a population growth out of control. "No despot ever flung forth his legions to die in foreign conquest," declared Margaret Sanger, founder of Planned Parenthood, in 1920. "No privilege-ruled nation ever erupted across its borders, to lock in death embrace upon another, but behind them loomed the driving power of a population too large for its boundaries and its natural resources. No period of low wages or of idleness with their want among workers, no peonage or sweatshop, no child-labor factory, ever came into being, save from the same source" (3). Clearly influenced by evolutionary theory and the new movement of eugenics that borrowed from it, Sanger understood the limitations to natural resources to be a strain on the survival of a growing population. Purposely inhibiting maternity would both secure the borders of private property and curtail competition in the work force. While the new parameters of a culture of competition would now include women and immigrants, limits to motherhood, even in Sanger's feminist-oriented and politically justified work, seem to be the cornerstone of a new conception of competition based on the conviction that poverty arose because of natural restrictions in resource availability.

The idea of a rugged masculinity at the core of human adaptability and female selection propels an endless competition, of males with other males of their own kind, over a fertility always yet to be realized. Darwin himself explains sexual selection in 1871: "This form of selection depends not on a struggle for existence in relation to other organic beings or to external conditions, but on a struggle between individuals of one sex, generally the males, for possession of the other sex. The result is not death to the unsuccessful competitor, but few or not offspring.... Generally, the most vigorous males, those which are best fitted for their places in nature, will leave the most progeny. But in many cases, victory depends not so much on general vigor, as on having special weapons, confined to the male sex" (117). He further remarks that "individual males hav[e] had in successive generations, some slight advantage over other males, in their weapons, means of defense, or charms, which they have transmitted to their male offspring alone" (119). The processes through which evolution occurs creates a masculinity in defense against a threatened population extinction that female sexual abstinence invites. Survival depends on the successful and efficient overcoming of such barriers to copulation, where female withdrawal creates a demand for increasing male competition and the development of superior qualities to overcome it.

Darwin produced sterility as a central focus of evolutionary researches by centralizing sex as a transformative but slow and gradual principle working in conjunction with environmental alterations to create diversity in biological systems. Before Darwin, the essence of species was considered, though problematically and with much contention, to be contained within reproductive family lines. Species either could not cross and continue to reproduce, or they could only reproduce sterile offspring; they were, by definition, reproductively segregated. In the early nineteenth century, Sir Charles Lyell's popular theory of "uniformitarianism" (*Principles of Geology* [1830]), for instance, professed that there was not enough evidence in the fossil record to prove species transformation, that all change could be accounted for by processes still in operation, and that therefore individuals within a species "have certain distinguishing characters in common, which will never vary, and which have remained the same since the creation of the species" (12). In his famous 1865 paper "Experiments in Plant Hybridization," the so-called father of genetics, Gregor Mendel, concentrated his experiments on crossing plants of the same species and counting the recurrences of certain well-defined traits like color or texture. His conclusions showed that recessive traits could reappear in successive generations of the same species, proving the stability of species essence as well as the unlikelihood of biological change within a species.[7] Later in the century, Darwin's cousin Francis Galton, the founder of statistics and the eugenics movement, believed that species, when crossed, tended to revert to their parent forms, or toward the population "norm" at the tip of the bell curve, because features did not blend.

Based on his observations of domestic breeding, Darwin was able to reevaluate reproduction between species and reformulate the reproductive boundaries by which species had been categorically contained.[8] "We must, therefore," Darwin asserted in *Origin of Species*, "either give up the belief of the universal sterility of the species when crossed; or we must look at this sterility in animals, not as an indelible characteristic, but as one capable of being removed by domestication" (370). Before there was an adequate theory of genetics to account for trait transmissions, sex, for Darwin, would provide the setting for evolutionary transformations and special change by mixing traits.

In page after page, natural selection is nothing if not a grueling and detailed display of sex and its controls, where the controls are variously shifting from environmental depletion to female scarcity. Darwin's thinking on the relationships between environment and reproduction changed between *Origin of Species* and *The Descent of Man. Origin* sets up a relationship between environment and reproduction wherein many sets of variables are at work to keep an unsteady ecological balance; female reproduction plays only a small part in the many possibilities of life and selection. Compressing this multifaceted explanation into a perennially repeatable sex story, Darwin's development of a theory of sexual selection in *Descent*, meanwhile, foregrounds female sexual constraint as the principal manifestation of resource limitation, the principal reason for competition, the principal catalyst for adaptation and transformation, and, therefore, the principal mechanism for survival. Now centered within a singular narrative of sterility, female sexuality became the metaphoric backbone for a host of environmental activities and limitations, causes and controls, which were formerly brought into play through vast networks of interconnected environmental, economic, and population pressures.

Evolution, as Darwin envisions it in *Origin*, set up reproduction as a product of an initial scarcity. Darwin conceived his theory of the struggle for existence as a competition to reproduce as much as the particular, local environment would allow. The available food supplies were limited by environmental factors, such as seasonal variation and the proximity of competitors within the region: "The action of climate seems at first sight to be quite independent of the struggle for existence; but in so far as climate chiefly acts in reducing food, it brings on the most severe struggle between the individuals, whether of the same or of distinct species, which subsist on the same kind of food" (96). Reproduction enters the picture as a ratio of population increase, which puts added pressure on the food supply. The species that are checked by environmental limits and reproductive controls are favored by nature, as too great a rate of increase would diminish the chances for survival within a limited ecological niche. "A struggle for existence," Darwin said, "inevitably follows the high rate at which all organic beings tend to increase. Every being, which during its natural lifetime produces several eggs or seeds, must suffer destruction during some period of its life, and during some season or occasional year, otherwise, on the principle of geometrical increase, its numbers would quickly become so inordinately great that no country could support the product" (91). The variable rates of reproduction in a species, in a certain geographical milieu, are in proportion to the seasonal variation in the availability of food resources and the competition over them. Darwin here even elides the concept of resource depletion into an idea about government itself being victimized or challenged by the pressures of overpopulation, suggesting that imperial rule has been weakened.

Evolution happens, then, through shortages in ecobiological systems, shortages that lead to periodic destruction in order to make room for population. "This geometrical tendency to increase must be checked," says Darwin, "by destruction at some periods of life" (93). Whereas Darwin starts defining what he means by destruction by describing a cataclysmic event, a rapid decrease in stock or a sudden large-scale population reduction, he immediately switches to a laborious vignette about slow breeders who, even under favorable circumstances, "require more years to people . . . a whole district" (93). The image of a huge environmental explosion with countless deaths slips into an explanation of beneficial checks in population growth based on "those [organisms] which produce few [eggs or seeds]" (93). Like starvation, reproduction *is* a *natural* mode of destruction: a population control and a catastrophic sign of maximum environmental density, an economic strain. Evolution depends on death to keep the balance. The causes of death are natural rather than social. The environment selects those who learn to survive within it most aptly, while killing off those who are not suited, and all this to everybody's benefit. The environment—rather than stresses on certain populations owing to business speculation, low industrial wages, urban blight, factory conditions, and insecure property holdings—dictates the terms for survival.

One of the many causes of limited reproductive rates is a failure in the reproductive outcome of the male's attempts, through courtship and seduction, to create survival conditions within the fertilization process. "There must sometimes be a physical impossibility in the male element reaching the ovule, as would be the case with a plant having a pistil too long for the pollen-tubes to reach the ovarium" (381). Or, Darwin continues, the surface of the female body might itself resist penetration. Even if there is success in this initial contact, a number of obstacles might come into play as the narrative enters into more advanced stages on the path to reproduction. These additional obstacles are cataclysmic and destructive elements within the female reproductive system. The embryo might perish early or late in utero, or at an early stage of maturation, because of an insufficiency in the nutritive conditions within the mother's womb, for example. The environmental checks through which natural selection operates are replicated as an imbalance within the mother's womb, making male reproductive success as difficult, hazardous, and competitive a process as is the competitive hunt for food.

Darwin's contributions to the study of biology were largely derived from his interest in agricultural breeding. Two of the main innovations in Darwin's evolutionary researches and experimentation were therefore borrowed from the long-time practices of breeders: domestication and hybridization. "Domestication" involves breeding a plant in an environment where it is not indigenous for the purposes of controlling its outcome, traits, or rates of fertility; "hybridization" is the process of cross-breeding species, often by introducing strains with which the plants might not come into natural contact. "I have more than once," Darwin noted, "alluded to a large body of facts showing that, when animals and plants are removed from their natural conditions, they are extremely liable to have their reproductive systems seriously affected. . . . Between the sterility thus superinduced and that of hybrids, there are many points of similarity" (383). Both these concepts, as experimental ground rules, were about simulating environmental conditions to see how organisms would react to artificial change and controlled spaces. They were also based on the idea that sex was the cornerstone of any transformative process in special development, and so needed to be both observed and manipulated. While domestication, on the one hand, refers to the imposition of spatial boundaries on the extension of available resources, hybridization, on the other, signified the reproductive boundaries that could be artificially induced in controlled situations. Darwin's linking of these two methods served to show how environment and reproduction were, inextricably and interchangeably, part of the same process of controlling population growth in a world of scarcity.

The domestication of plants was what first allowed Darwin, according to his own account in *Origin of Species*, to understand the role of the environment in producing the economic conditions necessary for variability and special diversity. On this basis, Evelleen Richards has argued how Darwin's theory of natural selection was a metaphoric re-enactment of Victorian ideals of domesticity. Richards argues that Darwin's theory was based on the idea that civilization could be measured by the degree and extent of sexual difference, and therefore was seeped in the Victorian ideologies of separate spheres: "As the breeder selects and shapes his domestic productions so man has moulded woman to his fancy.... In the case of human selection, Darwin identified the human male with the breeder—... he put into men's hands the modifying and shaping power of the breeder" (78). In fact, it is difficult to pin down the origin of authority in Darwin's ideas on natural selection. In some sense, reproduction itself dictates the creative terms of survival. As Gillian Beer argues, "The natural order produces itself, and through reproduction it produces both its own continuance and its diversity. [Darwin's] theory had no place for an initiating nor intervening creator" (53). Margot Norris elaborates:

> While in the beginning of the *Origin of Species* Darwin stressed the breeder's power to modify and alter domestic breeds of plants and animals radically, in *The Variation of Animals and Plants under Domestication,* published almost a decade later, he took pains to dismantle the eugenicist's role. He did so by pointing out that the natural process remains independent of the breeder, who can control its direction but not its workings, and whose intervention will therefore have the same effect whether it is conscious or unconscious, voluntary or involuntary.... The breeder *imitates* natural selection. When he culls the inferior members of a herd and destroys the weaklings to prevent their reproduction, he *imitates,* consciously or unconsciously, the action of animal predators. (44–45)

What is clear is that domestication in evolutionary theory does not secure a male position of authority but actually destabilizes it, subjecting the authority of the breeder to checks through natural processes and reproductive failures at least partially outside of controls. Considering the metaphoric association—in metaphysical and philosophical traditions and even now, in the New Age consumer market—between woman and nature, such natural possibilities for jeopardizing evolutionary processes might lead to a call—perhaps in violence, perhaps in production—for a tighter-fisted, instrumental manipulation of women and nature. Darwin's theory of domestication actually expresses a nostalgia for reasserting a central authority while showing how other forces are contending with it.

Domestication would provide the closest possible replication of the model of geographical isolation found on the Galapagos Islands, where large amounts of natural immigration could not affect the ecostructure or the competitive balance and where the availability of food was limited by natural boundaries. Domestication, however, was not natural but an artificial environmental change that often seriously, even permanently, affected reproductive systems. "When, on the one hand," Darwin recounted,

> we see domesticated animals and plants, though often weak and sickly, breeding freely under confinement; and when, on the other hand, we see individuals, though taken young from a state of nature perfectly tamed, long-lived and healthy . . . , yet having their reproductive system so seriously affected by unperceived causes as to fail to act, we need not be surprised at this system, when it does act under confinement, acting irregularly, and producing offspring somewhat unlike their parents. (26–27)

Darwin used domestication, as a model for a much slower-moving environment in perpetual shift, to study the ways an environment in flux, with limited resources, would influence reproduction. For Darwin, domestication was a place where reproduction was kept in perpetual suspense, with sterility allowing the time-gaps for a narrative of development and transformations. As a small-scale model, domestication showed how environment worked to produce sterility through altering reproductive affinities, and how such sterility could be partly overcome through developing alternative sexual characteristics.

One of the ways that breeders could artificially produce this condition of sterility was by mixing different species. The experimentation on which evolution was built tended to look at special crossing as a major key to understanding what caused new species to emerge through transformation. Evolutionary science then debated the significance of crossing in face of invalidating evidence and theological arguments that hybrids tended to revert to parental forms, or become sterile and then extinct. Harriet Ritvo (1996) has shown how hybridity was a major concern to naturalists and practitioners of animal husbandry throughout the nineteenth century.

Species, she says, were supposed to manifest a "preventive aversion" (39) toward one another, creating natural sexual boundaries. However, such boundaries, she continues, were not reliable; indeed, many people speculated on what would happen if such couplings took place. In particular, female animals became a problem because, even confined and controlled, their limited reproductive capacities made them able to obstruct and confuse the experimental designs of the breeders. Darwin, however, postulated that species and varieties were not so distinct, and that therefore there was a very gradual and ever so slight progression between species strains: "Many cases are on record," he says in *Origin*, "showing that a race may be modified by occasional crosses, if aided by careful selection of the individuals which present the desired character; but to obtain a race intermediate between two quite distinct races, would be very difficult" (39).

As a parallel structure to domestication, hybridity for Darwin was a natural eugenic device that produced constraints on fertility, allowing for the optimization of available resources by controlling population growth rates. It was beneficial because it allowed species to exist, grow, and reproduce in a limited environment strained by high competition, from its dense population, over its resources. Hybridity naturally restricted reproductive rates by creating partial or occasional sterility through systemic incompatibilities, noncorresponding features, nonconforming "periodical actions" (384), and "unknown differences in their reproductive systems" (378). "As in hybridization. . . ," Darwin asserted, "the capacity is limited by a systematic affinity. . . . But this capacity . . . is by no means absolutely governed by systematic affinity" (377). Hybridization acts as a limitation to population because female sexuality is periodically restricted and seasonally variable, creating incompatibility between species. Environmental heterogeneity recreates reproductive barriers as slippery, partial, and temporal.

In *The Descent of Man*, Darwin reduced these complicated ideas about natural selection into the much simpler metaphor of sexual selection. Sexual selection works on the basis that the entire field of competition over scarce resources—the checks on population put into play by both domestication and hybridization—could be encompassed by the singular mechanism of female choice. This model contends that females hold out for the better choice, and that males develop characteristics to please them, excelling in hunting, in fighting, or in aesthetic traits. Darwin's descriptions show that female choice depends on male displays, lures, and window-dressings. They position females as consumers of male baits and combative violences. A natural aesthetic taste allows females to discern the better and more beautiful choices for evolutionary fortitude:

> It has been shewn that the largest number of vigorous offspring will be reared from the pairing of the strongest and best-armed males, victorious in contests over other males, with the most vigorous and best-nourished females, which are the first to breed in the spring. . . . And this will especially hold good if the male defends the female, and aids in providing food for the young. The advantage thus gained by the more vigorous pairs in rearing a larger number of offspring has apparently sufficed to render sexual selection efficient. (221)

Darwin's idea was that secondary sex characteristics in males were signs of special adaptation and advancement. The entire field of complex environmental operations, where food scarcity gave rise to all sorts of population controls, here gets funneled into a narrative of courtship emerging from the singular cause of female sexual restraint and the desire for more.

In the case of *Descent,* for instance, hybridity results when the female prefers the attractions and charms of a male from another species. She is therefore willing to hold out for longer, and so males develop even more courageous and vigorous traits to pass down to their male offspring. "But hens," for example, "will often avoid the officious attentions of young males. Old hens, and hens of a pugnacious disposition, the same writer [Mr. Brent] informs me, dislike strange males and will not yield until well beaten into compliance. Ferugon, however, describes how a quarrelsome hen was subdued by the gentle courtship of a Shanghai cock" (417). Clearly, females would choose the males who have acquired the most congenial properties (if not the most strength with which to abuse them). Production is about beauty, and female consumption of beauty causes male acquisitions.

Ultimately, female choice is the groundwork and explanation for what becomes male evolutionary supremacy. Humanity is the only species where, in Darwin's rendering, the male has managed to become the agent of sexual selection. Through eons of acquiring characteristics that make him more rugged and vigorous through hunting and protecting, he has assumed the role of deciding with whom he will mate: "The strongest and most vigorous men,—those who could best defend and hunt for their families, who were provided with the best weapons and possessed the most property, such as a large number of dogs or other animals,—would succeed in rearing a greater average number of offspring than the weaker and poorer members of the same tribes. There can, also, be no doubt that such men would generally be able to select the more attractive women" (595).

Male supremacy is about property, and as much as dogs and animals, the acquisition of offspring through choosing the right female mates would assure the evolution of personal wealth. Female choice itself has made female powers of intelligence and survival weaker, subjecting them to periods of disuse where they have all but atrophied or disappeared. Because, for instance, males have had to use their intelligence to charm females with their prowess on the hunt, female intelligence has diminished. Since acquired characteristics are often transmitted to offspring of the same sex, giving girls a similar education to boys would not suffice to bridge the gap between the sexes, but instead girls would need "to be trained to energy and perseverance" (565) that could then be transmitted to their adult daughters. According to Darwin, female choice led to the increased sexual difference, which is a sign of civilized culture, but in the process, women have been left behind, punitively, guilty of having acquired excessive choosiness and wanting to be pleased too much.

Ever since the origin of a feminist movement in the Enlightenment, "choice" has been one of its dominant metaphors for political participation, from the struggle for suffrage to current advocacy for abortion rights. Mary Wollstonecraft, for example, imagines a feminism built through education: the "choice" of female political participation in the vote is defended because the discipline, morals, and virtue natural to women would acquire cultivation as they "exercise their minds" in rational engagement for the progress of civilization. By allowing "choice," knowledge, in Wollstonecraft's writings, would open the route toward equality between the sexes, improving practices of mothering, ensuring social health, fashioning women as citizens, and freeing human progress from the shackles of female dependency. However, as the politics of "choice" is—and has been since the Victorians—embedded in ideas about property ownership, economic depletion, hardship, and limited access, it might be advantageous to rethink how "choice" restricts the reach of a political agenda. In its current circulation, the term "choice" seems to imply the "choice" of consumer items or "lifestyles" based on the individual sovereignty—or independence—of a person with financial control or, within U.S. feminism, the "choice" of careers and professions, of an access to steady income. For example, when considering gender equity in the classroom, an unusually critical education textbook, *The Way Schools Work,* like many others, defines sexism as "discrimination against women, as in restricted career choices, job opportunities, etc." (259). The authors never even mention that, say, welfare cutbacks, inadequate health care, dirty water, civil wars, the lack of day care, or public schools without funding for textbooks affect female choices worldwide to a much greater degree than the restricted economic decision making of those who actually have the privilege of choosing such things as careers and defining this as progress. Feminism should not only be about economic assimilation. The idea of "choice" within feminism seems to confine both its theory and movement from pursuing a more global radical politics or, at the very least, goals that are not based solely on economic rationality, on a corporate mentality of competing on an even scale, on inclusion. World poverty, famine, violence against women, inner-city indigence, environmental destruction, political terror—these are not problems that stem naturally from the limitations of the world economy and for the need to make a "choice" about allocations of jobs and things, but rather direct effects of capitalist exploitation, the *lack* of restrictive controls on corporate production, the *unmitigated* spread of markets and consumer ideas, the disproportioning of *profuse* financial power, the unjust accumulation of some at the expense of others. Perhaps the centrality of "choice" within feminism conceals the international class struggle and the natural abundance of a world in production. And perhaps feminism would do better to think along these lines.

In sexology, psychology, and later in psychoanalysis, the play between female sexual restraint and environmental deficiencies continued to operate as evolution surfaced inside definitions of femininity and of female sexualities. In such evolutionary paradigms, female scarcity still instigated a narrative delay in which male competition was configured as the baseline principle of genetic survival and perfectibility. Necessary for marking the increasing intelligence of humanity and the moral superiority defining the white race, female infertility, within nineteenth-century studies of sexuality, got centered as the vortex through which evolutionary stories were told. The study of psychology developed further the idea, in both evolutionary science and economics, that society was composed of individualized figures devoid of outside forces like the cultural logic of consumption, making decisions on the margins. Female choice provided the narrative line in which could be justified and exhibited a rationality-in-production, the humanization of an independent agency in the process of deciding, thinking, and choosing from a display of beautiful things and attractions in competition.

As evolutionary paradigms were adopted into studies of psychology, the continuing dominance of competition, acquisition, choice, restriction, and persistent need as explanations of human behavior marks debt—or lack—as an economic concept central to individuation. What is dangerous in this psychologically individuated subject is the virtual insularity of the subject in most narratives of development, where social forces, such as schooling or poverty, injustice or inequality, are absent from studies, understandings, and explanations of behavior. Yet, fixed outside of economic influences, the subject in psychoanalysis is still born out of the natural desire to consume and the impossibility of realizing that desire, the subject propelled toward progress by the constant negation of achieving it. In particular, Freud himself based his psychoanalytic studies on the concept of female scarcity that had already been carried over from evolutionary biology into the fields of sexology and psychology.

Borrowing from evolutionary biology the theory of recapitulation to explain individual maturation, psychology individualized the evolutionary process by recreating it as a developmental narrative of the mind.[9] Recapitulation stated that individuals repeated ancestral development during the course of growth. Freud's references to recapitulation sweep through many levels of his theories on how the psyche was structured. His catalogue of the perversions in *Three Essays on the Theory of Sexuality* (1905) pointed to various erotogenetic zones—the mouth, for example, whose oral excitation (in thumbsucking and other activities) remains behind from an earlier phase: from a primitive, cannibalistic search for nourishment—each superseded, in the linear course of development, until the final stage, where genital sexuality predominates as the sign of civilization. The Oedipal complex, too, moves in its complicated formations toward its final resting place in the superego's institution of conscience, the internalization of social regulation. The superego represents the culmination of development in the internalization of a punitive voice of denial: the voice of the father in the superego; the voice of loss that denies the boy's access to his mother, is left over, says Freud, from the glacial period:

> If we consider once more the origin of the super-ego as we have described it, we shall recognize that it is the outcome of . . . the lengthy duration in man of his childhood helplessness and dependence, and the fact of his Oedipus complex, the repression of which we have shown to be connected with the interruption of libidinal development by the latency period and so with the diphasic onset of man's sexual life. According to one psycho-analytic hypothesis, the last-mentioned phenomenon, which seems to be peculiar to man, is a heritage of the cultural development necessitated by the glacial epoch. (1960, 31)

The unmet demands of the hungry child and the primitive ancestor cause the superego's formation of guilt as the highest form of civilization. Like the economic consumer, which is formed out of desires for what it cannot have, the superego rises as a subject-in-want, struggling to compensate, to acquire.

In psychology, female sexuality—its delays, its modesties, and its periodic lacks of impulse—was a principal cause of hunger and shortage. The conception of psychology that emerged in the nineteenth century relied on the centrality of female infertility, scarcity, and delay so integrated within an evolutionary model. It linked female rhythms to environmental factors, where females seasonally turn away from sex when nutrients are low in supply, and imagined masculinity as developing ingenuity and efficiency for the purposes of reproductive success. Havelock Ellis, for example, placed the periodic nature of female desire at the heart of his scientific studies on human sexuality. Only in summer, Ellis contends for example, are does in rut, when enormous expenditures of energy, increased metabolism, and musculatory build-up develop from sexual pursuit. "If a doe dislikes the attention of a special buck, miles of racing result," he writes. "If jealous males meet, furious battles take place. The strain on both sexes could not possibly be endured at any other season of the year" (1901, I, P. 1: 125). When the food supply is plentiful, females will sexually engage. The periodic and seasonal patterns of female sexual disinterest among species in a state of nature explain evolution and human biological advances through male competition, conquest, acquisition, and eminence. However, Ellis does not mention, for instance, the role of industry or colonial trade policy in restricting the access to subsistence of some or giving the advantage to others to win the chase.

In "The Evolution of Modesty," the first chapter of his enormous collection of sex research, Ellis links female modesty to animal periodicity in order to show its basis in nature: "We have found among the factors of modesty . . . the primitive animal gesture of sexual refusal on the part of the female, when she is not at that moment of her generative life at which she desires the male's advances" (80). Such reclusiveness on the part of the female leads to various strategies on the part of the male, which, in turn, engender civilized social life, such strategies, for example, as ritual practices, rules of decorum, the Muslim veil, and the institution of marriage as a form of property containment:

> It is doubtless the necessity for this probationary period, as a test of masculine qualities, which usually leads a woman to repel instinctively a too hasty and impatient suitor, for, as Arthur Macdonald remarks, "It seems to be instinctive in young women to reject the impetuous lover, without the least consideration of his character, ability, and fitness." This essential element in courtship, this fundamental attitude of pursuer and pursued, is clearly to be seen even in animals and savages; it is equally pronounced in the most civilized men and women. (41)

Modesty eventually breaks down as men rise to the challenge. "The immense importance of feminine modesty in creating masculine passion must be fairly obvious" (1), he proclaims. In Ellis's conception, social behavior is locked into the natural and the biological: the laws of nature determine the way social institutions and behavioral conventions form. Based on a model of environmental scarcity, female modesty represents a test-case scenario for fundamental masculine ingenuity and individual, physical transcendence marking the evolution of civilization.[10]

In their 1889 study *The Evolution of Sex,* Patrick Geddes and J. Arthur Thomson envisioned reproduction as an evolved form of the hunt for food, and sexual difference as conforming to the anabolic and katabolic functions: "The union of sperm with egg results when the hungry sperm pursues the egg as a source of nourishment; the egg, being amply supplied with food, is less disposed to the chase" (Mosedale; 36). The female is passively nutritive, waiting for the male to expend enough energy because of environmental demands and the subsequent rise in appetite. Likewise, sexologist James Kiernan equated sexual desire to appetite because sexual union has evolved from the metabolic functions of cannibalistic amoeba: "Hence, it is that the small starving male seeks out the larger well-nourished female for purposes of conjugation, to which the latter, the larger and better nourished, is on its motive less inclined" (190). Females are simply less hungry. The diminishment of the sexual appetite, which in Kiernan's schema is one explanation for inversion, is sometimes caused by things such as "tribal customs" (204), morbid cannibalism (199), living "several years among the Indians" (203), or "conditions in lower and even in primitive forms" (199).

Freud, too, worked out a theory of sexuality and development based on periodic female scarcity within an ecological model. Freud's cartographies of human development, with their narratives of scarcity, are modeled on evolutionary biology's central story of periodic female sexual unavailability representing low food supplies within an environmental niche. Freud conceived of his Oedipal theory during his correspondence, in the 1890s, with Wilhelm Fleiss, who was, at the time, positing a law of biological periodicity based on bisexuality. For Fleiss, evolution had interposed a female cycle onto a male cycle as the foundation of an original bisexual disposition. The female cycle proceeds from a periodic depletion of nutritive energy that was expended in the male cycle. Freud's first papers were on the bisexual nature of the nervous system of the arcadians, whose male features replenished the depletions of the female cycle (Sulloway, 159).

The Oedipal crisis is predominantly a narrative borrowed from evolutionary biology showing the maturation of the mind through a crisis of scarcity. Through the romance of Oedipus, the little boy's arrival into the social, sexual, and symbolic networks of adulthood is already mediated through competition with the father for the mother, a competition that must ever be waged but can never be won. Access to the mother is denied to the little boy, and his entire mental life derives from the unmet desire that ensues. In castration, the inaccessibility of the mother becomes a source of panic for the little boy. He sees what he cannot have and becomes a subject in want.

Following on Lévi-Strauss's work on kinship, Marxists feminists in the 1970s and 1980s used psychoanalysis to show how women entered networks of alliance as objects of exchange. In "The Traffic in Women," for example, Gayle Rubin argues that through the exchange of women, men enlarged their social and symbolic associations, just as through the gift, in Marcel Mauss's work, the giver initiates a permanent relation of reciprocity with the receiver of the gift. Like these anthropological models, the Oedipal cycle forms social institutions and alliances through the circulation of women, but unlike these other models, psychoanalysis uses the circulation of women to talk about a fundamental scarcity at the heart of mental functioning, the constriction of desire as a founding moment. Like the environment in evolution, psychoanalysis considers the mind as insular, a stable thermodynamic unit whose interacting forces are uniform and predictable within an enclosed niche—the family.[11]

In Freud, nervous diseases, constitutional disorders, neuroses and psychoses, indicated, for the most part, reversions to ancestral moments of periodically limited sexual instinct in women. In his notes from 1915 on transference neuroses, Freud recognized female hysteria as a regressive condition resulting from a conflict between the instinct for self-preservation in a world of scarce resources and the desire, linked to the death instinct, to procreate. Freud (1987) tells of a time of originary abundance, when the environment, a "primeval paradise" (13), was rich enough to satisfy all needs. The recurrence of hysterical symptoms, for Freud, was a recapitulation of the overturning of this earlier stage of plenitude where primal humanity "may have overcome the periodicity of the libido, which is still connected in mammals" (13). The subsequent coming of the Ice Age caused a depletion in the availability of resources, and a resulting "social obligation to limit reproduction . . . affect[ing] women more severely than men" (15) because "the powers of the individual were not adequate to keep so many helpless beings alive" (14). Environmental limitations caused the division between the sexes, which came to mark the foundation of the social contract leading to civilized governance. Repressing their desire, men then developed methods of rerouting libidinal activities into superior cultural and intellectual endeavors.

For Freud, the Oedipal complex recreates the struggle over resources in the glacial period as a specifically gendered contract. The Oedipal scene, in fact, divides gender according to the economic principles of material plenty and lack, where the sexed position of "man" is in constant struggle to retain what an economy of exchange is threatening to take away. In *Totem and Taboo* (1913), the primal horde of sons, introducing the cycle, slaughters and then eats the father because he would not let them touch his women. Replacing the threat of the Ice Age (with its depletion of resources), the primal father and then the law of the brothers are now what prohibit access to women—"No males to touch the females in my camp" (126)—laying the foundations for sociability in the horde. The Oedipal crisis, where the son competes with the father—"Some cultural advance, perhaps, command over some new weapon, had given ... a sense of superior strength" (141–42)—over access to the mother—"the sons acknowledged their father's sexual privilege by renouncing all claim to their mother and sisters" (142)—represents the catalyst to culture, religion, morality, ritual, and community at the origin of civilization. As primary, prohibatory taboos limiting access to women, food, and things, monogamy and the feast become the founding institutions of social living.

Such limited availability of women in ancestral cultures is the model on which Freud constitutes all psychic life. This normalized, foundational narrative of human mental development in males twists into an explanation for the etiology of disease, aberration, abnormality, and, in particular, hysteria in women. According to Freud's analysis of Dora (1905), his patient's repressed memory is set as her flight from Herr K.'s sexual advances. "The question arises," Freud comments in a footnote, "If Dora loved Herr K., what was the reason for her refusing him in the scene by the lake? Or at any rate, why did her refusal take such a brutal form, as though she were embittered against him? And how could a girl who was in love feel insulted by a proposal which was made in a manner neither tactless nor offensive?" [31]. The central spin of Dora's case is her rejection of Herr K., from which point the entire developmental narrative of her sexuality and neurosis proceeds. By making herself inaccessible, Dora initiates a course of desire that spurs, as Freud concludes, the man's "heroic exploits, all his successes . . . for the purpose of pleasing a woman" (113–14). The hazards and nutritional deficiencies implicated in the Ice Age story, through which men develop the institutions of civilization, are routed into a symbolism of psychic (hetero)sexual inhibition in women.

Freud explains female homosexuality as a shortage in female libidinal investment resulting in frustrated male desire, an arrest in the evolutionary progress of men, and therefore representing a male failure to attract and lure women in reproductive contests leading to hereditary transmissions of superior qualities. The love triangles set up in Dora's story, where two men vie for the attentions of one woman who plays hard to get and, in the end, turns away, implicate the corruption of male hereditary value; empty of the traits necessary for wooing and winning the affections of a mate, the idea of male inheritance is, in the case of Dora, fundamentally diseased, degenerative, and perverse: "Syphilis in the male parent is a very relevant factor in the aetiology of the neuropathic constitution of children" (14), notes Freud of Dora's father. In fact, Freud explains Dora's disgust at Herr K.'s kiss as a repugnance at her own venereal disease that both she and her mother contracted and that she believes was her father's fault, her constitutional heritage (67).

The lack of female engagement—the inaccessibility of women for male conquest—leads to developmental inertia with its contingent neurotic symptoms. In "A Case of Paranoia Running Counter to the Psychoanalytical Theory of the Disease" (1915), Freud defines psychic fixation and female sexual disinterest as an overdetermined desire between the female patient and her mother. "The mother thus becomes the hostile and jealous watcher and persecutor," Freud explains, a barrier to seduction. The bond between Dora and her mother, through which Freud detects a "homosexual current," stands in for the primitive barrier by which the law of the father, and then of the brothers, made women exclusively inaccessible. Like Dora's later affections for Frau K., Dora's identification with her mother removes her from a sexual circulation in which men would contend for her attentions. After all, she can only have a fake child, a mimetic one: nine months after the scene with Herr K. by the lake, Dora contracts appendicitis. Freud diagnoses Dora's appendicitis as "a phantasy of childbirth" (95). Prohibiting sexual access to her, her very body becomes the pronounced physiological site of her sexual barriers and restrictions.

Emerging historically in the lap of industrialization, psychoanalysis positions material lack as the motivation for human progress and thought. It is thereby instrumental in constructing a culture of interest consumerism. Gender divides producers and consumers into different spheres of interest and different types of life activities, all naturally proceeding toward a common good. Yet, such a politics based on "lack" justifies the demonization of, say, African-American women, who supposedly suck dry an economy that does not have enough to spare. It is true that desire and lack are the basis for political movements, even oppositional ones. Yet, the idea of scarcity that propels politics needs to be thought as motivated and controlled by historical agents who have everything to gain from such global assumptions that, say, the government is spending too much of a tax base which cannot support such spending. What produces scarcity is not a general depletion of resources nor a need for federal belt-tightening at a time of national crisis, deficit expansion, the contraction of the tax base, governmental overcommitment, or the lamentable national wailing about the next generation of unborn children inheriting our debt. Certainly, for example, scarcity does not explain the U.S. motivation to increase the military in preparation for two full-scale engagements and then some, or the gruesome displays of new technologies of air power—twenty-one spanking-new B-52 bombers star-spangling the skies over Kosovo, a $44 billion project brought to you by Northrop Grumman Corporation—and weapons of destruction under the banner of "bombs for peace." What is in evidence here is, rather, an abundance of production controlled by some at the expense of others, or, in other words, the distribution of scarcity as a mechanism to consolidate power and to support a culture of excessive spending, a culture that destroys the excess in an orgy of consumption.

Appendum: Strange Bedfellows

In August 1999, the Kansas state board of education struck the teaching of evolutionary theory out of the required curriculum for public schools.[12] The outcry in the national press was immediate. Supporters contended that the decision that evolution should not be included as mandatory material had less to do with Christianity's investments in creationism than with the status of evolutionary theory as an unprovable theory rather than a universal fact. Yet, undoubtedly, the events in Kansas participate in a tradition of conflict between evolution and creationism that marks the institutional boundaries between scientific objectivity and professions of faith in the interests of shoring up the power of both. Meanwhile, retractors challenged the decision on the grounds of the constitutional separation of church and state, or that Kansas students would then be noncompetitive in college application pools across the nation. The event became a high-exposure media spectacle, with much greater currency than, for instance, the Kansas state board of education's decision in 1998 to review all public school curriculum so that it could censure any "gay and lesbian content." The state board of education was moved in both instances by religious concerns, particularly its desire to impose Christian fundamentalist views on the entire state's population. But as Stephen Jay Gould protested, "We should cringe in embarrassment that, at the dawn of a new, technological millennium, a jurisdiction in our heartland has opted to suppress one of the greatest triumphs of human discovery" (1999: 59). Evolution has actually been observed and documented to a very large degree. Such efforts as this initiative in Kansas need to be resisted on every level; they are detrimental and even destructive to the principles of democracy.

Yet, why would such a story spark so much interest? After all, the decision on a state level does not necessarily mean that the policy will be implemented on a district level, for many of the local districts in Kansas have kept evolution on the agenda. Moreover, as the 1998 decision shows, the public school curriculum is often a site where various interests struggle over meaning and is often controlled by bureaucracies in ways that go against the public interest. The state board of education in Texas, for instance, controls the production of elementary school textbooks. When I was working on a spelling series for a big-league publisher, I was instructed that I could not include words like "jack o' lantern" because they promoted Satan worship and would therefore displease the Texas PTA, and displeasing the Texas PTA meant a certain commercial failure for the project. A colleague was working on a social studies series that was criticized by the Texas PTA on the grounds that the photographs in the books included too many faces of color and so did not accurately reflect the racial composition of either Texas or the nation. If the cutting of ideas and texts from public school curricula is happening frequently, without notice, why at this moment in history does a story of evolution become such an obsession that it is universally covered in the media and *Time* magazine features a cover story on it? What is at stake in evolutionary theory now?

Evolution tells a story about competition, and the story it tells about competition supports another story about market freedoms and the nature of unregulated competition. While most people think, *Time* begins, that evolution happened as a series of consecutive steps marking progress, there were in fact other human species that died out along the way. *Time* describes evolution as "an elimination tournament" where "all were competitors in an evolutionary struggle from which only one would ultimately emerge" (Lemonick and Dorfman, 52). *Homo sapiens* became the dominant survivor because these humans acquired traits that helped them adapt: bipedalism, toolmaking (which led to an increased capacity for meat-eating), and the growth of the brain (a power "which quickly led to art, music, language and all the other skills that have enthroned humans as the unchallenged rulers of their planet" [52] and happened simultaneously with the emergence from Africa). *Time* uses scenes of carnage to describe how these humans gained advantages by meat-eating, for instance, an antelope's jawbone with the tongue cut out or a carcass with the bones bashed open, evidencing signs of hammering. These scenes depict humans as emerging victorious in a competitive field because they had mastery of technologies of violence and could thus win out over their neighbors in a constant struggle for "an energy rich, high-fat diet" (57). The evolutionary tale naturalizes violent competition. Ethics, community, and compassion wane under more compelling carnivorous urges and ruthless contests for quick-profit protein growth at any cost. Innovation in (quite literally) cutting-edge technologies promises symbolic innovations as well: the production of superior art and lifestyles—"Art, symbols, music, notation, language, feelings of mystery, mastery of diverse materials and sheer cleverness" (58)—depends upon the protein consumption, brain growth, and the consequent creation and proliferation of tools for chopping up bodies.

In a post-Kosovo world, this popular representation of evolution deifies killing technologies, celebrating them as the very defining element of what it means to be "civilized," culturally and racially superior in evolutionary terms. The idea that global capitalist consolidation constitutes power is wiped out as the development of such technologies is attributed to a natural evolutionary musculature. Yet, the features of these evolutionary scenes certainly resemble much of the popular media's investigations into the phenomenon of globalization. For example, one of *homo sapiens'* competitors' remains was found with its skull badly crushed, says *Time,* probably because a hippo or an elephant stepped on it. The magazine's comment on the incident—"'It looks like roadkill,' quips [the archaeologist] White"—uncannily parallels *New York Times* correspondent Thomas Friedman's portrait of the global market, where "those who don't [perform] are left as roadkill on the global investment highway" (214). Such pundits use the law of nature as evidence that "those cultures that are not robust enough ... will be wiped out like any species that cannot adapt to changes in its environment" (236), instead of indicating that consolidated capital makes competition obsolete by allowing the powerful to control commercial infrastructures. "We cannot hope," continues Friedman, "to preserve every culture in the world just as it is.... As with species, cultures spawning, evolving and dying is part of evolution" (244). In this view, globalization results from processes of reproduction—what he calls "the procreation cycle," where consistently masculinized companies become agents of flirtation, and power emerges out of a series of successful seductions. Such globalization theories use popular conceptions of evolution to explain power as natural rather than tied to enormous financial advantages, which are certainly far from natural and which determine the outcomes of much of what passes as "free competition."

The Kansas story was not the first nor the last evolutionary tale to make its way into the popular media recently. National Public Radio has covered the archaeological excavations of the Leakeys' daughter as she returned to Olduvai Gorge to recommence the search for the missing evolutionary link. Archaeologists Louis and Mary Leakey had discovered *homo habilis* skeletal remains in Olduvai Gorge in the 1960s, and their son, Richard, had continued the search. But two weeks after the report on Kansas, *Time* again broached the topic of evolution as resulting from natural greed and the propensity to accumulate. Orangutans, for example, have the ability to calculate costs and profits and to manipulate astute deals in bartering situations. "[The orangutan] Colo opened his hand," *Time* cutely attests,

> and revealed that he was holding a key chain, much in the manner that a fence might furtively show a potential customer stolen goods on the street. Relieved that it was not anything dangerous or valuable, Charlene gave Colo

> the piece of pineapple. Astute bargainer that he was, Colo then broke the key chain and gave Charlene a link, perhaps figuring, "Why give her the whole thing if I can get a bit of pineapple for each piece?" (Linden, 58)

Animal studies have shown, *Time* insists, that animals are naturally good at business but a business that is ruthlessly competitive, unethical, and conniving or, as *Time* admiringly says, with more of a propensity toward "devious behavior than in acts of cooperation or love" (59). In fact, the intelligence and rationality of apes, as they "outfox" humans by cheating and linguistic deception, proves the evolutionary superiority of a free-market system. As *Time* says, "Indeed, it has been easier to defeat communism than to get scientists to agree on what Washoe meant three decades ago when she saw a swan on a pond and made the signs for 'water bird'" (57). As orangutans naturally calculate value in objects, rationality marks evolutionary advancement. This rationality can be witnessed as the ability to undermine and outsmart competitors, first in escaping from cages and zoos and then in turning maximum profits through trickery. This rationality, however, can only arise in apes who are relatively satisfied; when they are hungry, their "appetites persistently overcame [their] reason" (60). In other words, the rich are much more likely to develop these rational, natural, competitive qualities than those who want more than they already have. Consequently, poor people do not act according to rules that are calculating, rational, and therefore deserving of human freedom.

The Kansas story participates in a broader public dialogue over exactly where the limits to the federal government's powers should be staked in an age of globalization. The Kansas decision reflects a recognized discrepancy in "social contract theory," which admits a fundamental contradiction or trade-off between the interests of the individual and the interests of the state. Further, Kansas contributes to an old controversy in the United States between whether individual states or the federal government should have the right to mandate. This debate is foundational in the United States, the very substance behind the drafting of the Constitution, and leading once to a civil war, when the states' rights platform was mobilized to support the institution of slavery, not freedom. Today, however, the tradition of states' rights has been rewritten as the very foundation of freedom, while its histories of oppression have been obliterated from national memory.

Thus, as Katha Pollitt has pointed out, Al Gore is reluctant to criticize Kansas, "saying that the decision to teach evolution should be left to local school boards" (10), thus repeating the current dogma that local governments know better what is good for local citizens. Gore leaves aside the raging national battles over standards and federal testing, policies that the administration he works for has instrumentalized, in order to show his backing for federal curtailment.[13] Kansas sanctifies that border beyond which the federal government cannot go in the name of individual liberties. By clearly demarcating the limits of federal power, Kansas foregrounds the economics of neoliberalism as a moral posture supporting a space of pure, individual freedom and choice. This is an alibi. It diverts attention away from the fact that most of the time, as Friedman admits, "too much government" means federal checks on business enterprise, capitalist trickery, and the unmitigated growth of U.S. corporations (defined as the path to "freedom") at the expense of social programs, equality, and justice.

As evolution becomes a mass media spectacle, it justifies capitalism in its current form, reproducing inequalities as natural rather than as institutional imbalances and giving ideological support for the consolidation of corporate power. The Kansas controversy is not, then, as Jonathan Zimmerman contends in *The New Republic,* simply the result of mistakes made by multiculturalist reformists and feminists who have taken cultural relativism to an extreme.[14] "Multicultural curricula, especially," attests Zimmerman, "are guilty of espousing the insidious idea that there is no single Truth; there is only your truth and my truth, both of which usually reflect our different races, ethnicities, and genders. When it comes to evolution, however, these single-minded absolutists [i.e., creationists like Jerry Falwell] start to sound just like the multiculturalists they abhor" (14). The controversy over evolution in the national media does not result from a liberal agenda insisting that all ideas be included as equal and that there is no determining focal point from which knowledge can be assessed. Not only is this contention racist and sexist in its faulting of multiculturalism, but it is also unfounded. Extremely few advocates for multiculturalism would consider all knowledge claims equally valid.

Rather, the spectacle professes a carefully constructed plot serving specific political interests. These stories of evolution uphold the freedom to compete. They also serve to legitimate a consensual center in U.S. politics by marginalizing the Christian right from the mainstream of the Republican Party. Evolutionary stories participate in wider public discourses exonerating the Republican Party from what is widely considered the Christian right's extremist agenda. Such public discourses range from the attack on the Christian right's not-for-profit status, the criticism of its church collections for political issues and candidates, and George W. Bush's refusal to take on its challenges or take a stand on abortion in his presidential campaign. On the one hand, this strategy to marginalize the Christian right could be seen as a smart electoral tactic, given that its socially conservative policies no longer seem widely popular even among conservatives.

On the other hand, the Christian right is currently one of the few loud voices in the national public forum that are speaking out against the excesses of free market capitalism and globalization. For example, *The Nation* reports that at the Iowa straw poll, Teamsters were congregating at Pat Buchanan's camp, "wildly applaud[ing]" his anti-corporatist, pro-labor rhetoric. Pat Buchanan, says *The Nation,* is "the *only* presidential candidate today standing before unionized workers and calling for tougher application of antitrust laws, for a possible lifting of the economic blockades of Cuba and Iraq, who calls NAFTA 'a sellout of Americans for the benefit of a lot of bankers,' who laments that 'we need a leader from any party who will stand up for working Americans against giant transnational corporations'" (Cooper, 15). Henry Giroux is right in maintaining that Pat Buchanan is calling here for a racially exclusive monoculturalism and espousing policies that enable "white Americans to 'take back' their country" (184). It is essential that much of the Christian right's agenda—their anti-abortionism, attacks on gays and lesbians, regressive nationalism, white supremacy, and, indeed, their moves to censor public school curricula—be confronted if not defeated. We must, however, recognize that widespread blaming of the Christian right in the media coverage of the Kansas story operates to marginalize the critique of capital. The culturalist and moralist emphasis in the widespread liberal challenge to fundamentalisms tends to white out the possibilities of an alternative materialist vision or redistributive scheme to emerge. Instead, the news coverage of the Kansas event makes the freedom of competition seem the most desirable freedom to strive for and to achieve, the only possible freedom for the future, as well as singularly and naturally triumphant.

As educators, political activists, curriculum advocates and others concerned with the politics of democracy seek to challenge Kansas's censorship of evolution from the curriculum, they should also rethink the politics of evolution and question the ways that evolution is used to justify neoliberal and fiscally conservative policies. Evolution should not be taught as a support for market ideology and militarization. This does not mean that scientific descriptions of nature need to be washed over in a moralistic cleansing. As Stephen Jay Gould tells us, "no factual discovery of science (statements about how nature 'is') can, in principle, lead us to ethical conclusions (how we 'ought' to behave) or to convictions about intrinsic meaning (the 'purpose' of our lives)" (59). Rather, popular representations of science need to be read critically and nonobjectively as already loaded with ideological content, and this content needs to be unraveled and rewritten in light of different types of evolutionary tales. Reflected in both animal behaviors and archaeological remains, cooperation, love, community, and indeed solidarity are certainly beneficial rather than nonadaptive to the advancement of human freedom.

Conrad's Closet

> *As we are continually meeting in cities women who are one-quarter, or one eighth, or so on, male . . . so there are in the Inner Self similar half-breeds . . .*
>
> —Charles G. Leland, "The Alternative Sex," London, 1904

Critics have debated, in relation to Joseph Conrad's 1913 novel *Chance*, whether or not Mrs. Fyne, the cross-dressing feminist who rescues the protagonist Flora from the evil manipulations of her governess, is a lesbian. For example, Wilfred Dowden describes Mrs. Fyne as an obvious "virago," more than a simple caricature of a suffragette, because of her "unnatural" relationship, an "almost lover-like attraction," to the "girlfriends" (150–51), and C. B. Cox contends that Mrs. Fyne is filled with a "lesbian fury" when she tries to obstruct Flora's marriage to her brother Anthony. In his introduction to *Chance*, Alfred Kazin writes, "Mrs. Fyne's vociferous feminism may conceal sexual designs on 'poor' Flora" (xi), and Adam Gillon agrees that "in *Chance*, the aggressively feminist Mrs. Fyne exhibits all the traits of a lesbian. Flora's elopement with [Anthony] Roderick provokes her wrath" (140). But Helen Rieselback counters that Conrad is simply reflecting, in Mrs. Fyne, "the 'masculine' role of the ideologue and political activist," with the girlfriends "probably only" satisfying her "need for disciples" (203).

What is it that these critics see? What attributes and meanings are they retrospectively recognizing as identifying "lesbian" desire? What I argue here is that such a controversy internalizes, without specifically acknowledging, the contentious space of definition that the term "lesbian" was undergoing at the time Conrad wrote this novel. Lesbian criticism has debated the contours and configurations of "lesbianism"'s entrance into discourse, concluding, for the most part, that the term introduced unspecificity into histories and narratives of identity. Lesbian historicism has been unsettled about where and how to recognize "lesbians" in source materials; nevertheless, theoretical perspectives have noted the beginning of the twentieth century as a controversial, salient, and pivotal time for determining the particularities of "lesbian" historical presence; at the moment that "lesbian" became, within British medical and legal discourses, a category marking a crisis in knowledge, a category of difference. Lillian Faderman has attributed the invention of the lesbian to nineteenth-century romantic friendships, the suspicions they aroused in the new science of sexology, and the consequent creation of social spaces for lesbian communities after World War I. Despite the interest intimacy between women was arousing in the scientific literature, however, lesbian theorists have observed an epistemological anxiety surrounding the cultural spaces where the category was brought into play. In a 1918 libel suit brought by Maud Allan, star of a contemporary performance of Oscar Wilde's play *Salome,* against Noel Pemberton-Billing, for example, Allan's crime of participation in the "cult of the clitoris" was proven in court, according to Jennifer Travis, in her confessed sexual knowledge. This was "a kind of knowledge," concludes Travis in her analysis of the case, "that one is not supposed to "know" (159). In 1921, when the category subsequently came up for possible parliamentary sanctions, Lord Desart, director of public prosecutions, consequently evoked "lesbian" identity as a prohibitive category lacking a referent: "You are going to tell the whole world that there is such an offence, to bring it to the notice of women who have never heard of it, never thought of it, never dreamt of it" (as cited in Hart, 3). During the same period, as George Chauncey, Jr. has documented, the medical model, changed from "inversion," a deviance in gender roles, to "homosexuality," an aberration in sexual object choice. Such a transformation resulted, concludes Chauncey, in an increasing area of doubt which the non-crossgendered but still "homosexual" woman, the woman playing the role of "wife," introduced into scientific speculations about women's sexuality at this time, adding an unspecifiable taboo against all women's intimacies and associations—including feminism—with one another. For the critics to see "lesbian" or "not lesbian" in *Chance,* they would have to be applying the term to an unknowable space in history, a space that did not yet have a name but also did not yet indicate a definable set of unified referential qualifications.

Chance, then, becomes, within the retrospective of critical analysis, a conflictual site for determining the contours and configurations of a "gender trouble" constitutive of a categorical labeling of the "lesbian." However, the instability in the meanings of gender that the term "lesbian" introduces through the criticism is foreshadowed, in Conrad's text, by the instability in the purity of racial distinctions that would anchor, so to speak, the authority of imperial narratives. The criticism itself acknowledges that, for instance, the governess' "sexual rage" against Flora, is represented "as if animal passions both of lust and fear, had suddenly welled up from underneath the superficial crust of civilization" (Cox, 121). *Chance* literalizes the realignments in gender, which, Lynda Hart remarks, are crucial to turn-of-the-century legislation around the term "lesbian": "The distinction that was being made between heterosexuality and homosexuality was . . . built on a prior division between white, middle-class women and other(ed) women: women of color and working-class women" (4). At the time, degeneracy theory was linking nonwhite racial identities to gender impurities and pathologies within a language of science becoming more and more systematized, embedded, and pervasive.[1] In an 1893 study, *La donna deliquente*, a foundational text for the new field of "criminal anthropology," Caesar Lombroso and William Ferrero, for instance, use gender inversion as "proof" of "atavism" in criminal women,[2] thus underscoring gender difference in women as a physiological sign of evolutionary advancement, the morality of the white race:

> Due also to it [atavism] is the virility underlying the female criminal type; for what we look for most in the female is femininity, and when we find the opposite in her we conclude as a rule that there must be some anomaly. And in order to understand the significance and the atavistic origin of this anomaly, we have only to remember that virility was one of the special features of the savage women. In proof I have but to refer the reader to the Plates opposite, taken from Ploss's work, where we have the portraits of the Red Indian and Negro beauties, whom it is difficult to recognise for women, so huge are their jaws and cheek-bones, so hard and coarse their features. And the same is often the case in their crania and brains. (112)

Sexological studies also assumed the lack of sexual difference in women, their virility, as a racial marker and a regressive state. Margaret Otis, for example, in a 1913 study of interracial romantic relations between girls in reform schools, stated that "the difference in color, in this case, takes the place of difference in sex.... One girl ... admitted that the colored girl she loved seemed the man, and thought it was so in the case of the others" (113–14).[3]

The text of *Chance* is obsessively concerned with a type of femininity that appears as an uncertain marker for the knowledge of racial identities. I discuss here Conrad's focalization of a Foucauldian-type epistemology of sexuality dependent, formatively, on stories of colonialism. As Ann Laura Stoler has remarked, the bourgeois bedroom and metropolitan domestic space, which Foucault put at the center and apex of Western subjectivities and the discourses of biopolitics, were "tied to notions of being 'European' and being 'white'" (1995: 11). However, Stoler goes on, the constructions of "whiteness," shored up in discourses of the bourgeois bedroom, were intertwined with the historical positioning of racial boundaries within colonial domestic arrangements. In this chapter I present *Chance* as reflecting the very historical problematic of subjectivity created by a specific crisis in femininity that colonial encounters in part occasioned. Against Marianna Torgovnick's thesis that in Conrad's novels, "miscegenation is simply not within the ken of the narrative; it it is a 'love that dare not speak its name'" (147), I claim that because miscegenation is a "love that dare not speak its name," the native woman is still a central—and anxious—focus in *Chance.* Mrs. Fyne, as well as the governess and Flora herself, are in some sense modeled on Conrad's earlier characterizations of racialized women in *Almayer's Folly* (1895) and *An Outcast of the Islands* (1896).

In *Chance,* Flora's infertility is connected to her colonial travels. Just as Nina, in *Almayer's Folly,* and Aïssa, in *An Outcast of the Islands,* create ambiguities in the institutions of white authority and economic legacies maintained in the reproduction of white masculinity, Flora poses the threat of restricted reproduction of ("white") imperial subjects. The enduring trace of colonial miscegenation creates disruptive effects in representations of white female sexuality, effects that, in the retrospective of critical analysis, are recognized as denoting a "lesbian" presence.

First published in the United States, *Chance* was the novel that won Conrad financial success and popular recognition. It was, as well, his first novel to be written specifically with an audience of women in mind, treating the conventional women's theme—romance. Most critics also agree that *Chance* was the novel precipitating Conrad's downfall as a novelist, showing the first signs of the mental and/or nervous illness that would infect and qualitatively diminish his literary production for the rest of his career. Edward Said says of *Chance*, "Even today, with the keen critical predisposition towards technical virtuosity for its own sake, no one can fail to notice the extraordinary fate that linked together what must be the most arid and technical of Conrad's works with his most dramatic success before the public" (1966: 64). The reason, critics claim, that *Chance* is less powerful than Conrad's more acclaimed works, such as *Heart of Darkness* (1899), *Lord Jim* (1900) and *Nostromo* (1904), is that Conrad here turns his focus from "politics" (a category that, presumably, would exclude feminism) to psychological and sentimental motifs. Proclaims Adam Gillon, "Betrayal, the leitmotiv of *The Secret Agent* [1907] and *Under Western Eyes* [1911], still looms large in these two novels [*Chance* and *Victory* (1915)], but they are, like most of Conrad's late fiction, devoted primarily to the exploration of the flawed human heart" (139).

The critical division in Conrad's opus between the earlier, more eclectic and political novels and stories, and the later, more popular fictions is further marked by the projected audience of women in *Chance*. The mass appeal of the romantic plot, with its melodrama and its linear narration, seems then to correspond in *Chance* to the construction of popular markets through the construction and targeting of women readers. "There is a clear link," remarks Scott McCracken, "between the overt concern for gender in *Chance* and its reputation as a 'down-market'" (279). Patricia Maria Feito notes that the division, as projected in *Chance*, between serious art and mass culture, is gender inflected.[4]

Frederic Jameson's developmental schema for the origins of modernism in Conrad poses a split and a dialectical convergence in Conrad's prose between a popular form of realist melodrama on the one hand, and aesthetic reflexivity, or literary impressionism, on the other, registering the emergence of a separate cultural space for "high" modernist discourse. According to Feito, the seeds of what Jameson, writing of Conrad in *The*

Political Unconscious, terms "the commercialized cultural discourse of what, in late capitalism, is often described as a media society" (206), reflects a broader strain within modernism of a crisis in authority brought about by a new problematics of gender: "If as Jameson argues, Conrad marks the beginnings of the break between realism and modernity, between that is, romance and impressionism, then *Chance*, I would argue, gives that problem a gender. It defines and contains the critical issues surrounding the emergence of modernism in England in terms of gender distinctions" (150). Certainly, Conrad himself, in *Chance*, makes such a distinction when he has Marlow say of the story, the "light literature" fairy tale, just told, "It is not exactly a story for boys" (246). There is a cheapness, a fakeness to such a world as women would create, Marlow imagines, a world "where the Irrelevant would fantastically step in to take the place of the sober humdrum Imaginative" (93). Such a creation, like "light literature," would be nondurable, easily breakable, a mere parody of the real creation, filled with empty and fragile clichés and "hackneyed illusions" (94). Arguing that Mrs. Fyne's feminist "form of Platonic academy for girls" puts her in the position of a Socrates-like philosopher, Feito suggests, for instance, that as Mrs. Fyne "steps into an arena under the surveillance of a powerful modern feminine subjectivity," she poses "a threat to masculine hierarchies simply by turning the objects of its domestic gaze into the subjects of writing," and so is converted into an "ethical monstrosity" (173). *Chance*, indeed, stages the confrontation between "high" and "low" culture as emerging through gender hierarchies, domestic conflicts, and the challenges posed by feminism.

Conrad's adoption of the conventions of realist romance, however, does not necessarily obliterate his earlier concern for a narrative critique of imperialism but instead displaces it. As Scott McCracken observes, "This absence [of the colonial subject in *Chance*] masks, more than is usual in Conrad's narratives, the centrality of the history of imperialism in the function of the ship, the *Ferndale*, which links up the global outposts of the British Empire" (277). For Jameson, too, the institutionalization of a "high literature" coexisting, in Conrad's tales, with earlier realisms corresponded to a partial repression "of a world of work and history and of protopolitical conflict" (207). The space of the sea, for example, Jameson describes as realism's "place of labor" (213) and a sign for the imperialist penetration of precapitalist zones. In *Chance*, the *Ferndale* symbolizes the site of domesticity and familial drama without ever completely escaping its role as a metaphoric gateway into imperialist governance and accessible industrial labor markets. What I am suggesting is that Conrad's exploration of gender relations in *Chance* is fashioned within a colonial historicism. Conrad's rendition of the New Woman, and of a female sexuality influenced by feminist doctrine, does not so much mask the history of colonialism nor absent it but rather secretly embodies it.

My argument here is that the symbolization of femininity in *Chance* both conceals and reveals underlying histories of colonial relations. I explore the ways in which mixed-race, colonized women, in Conrad's earlier novels *Almayer's Folly* and *An Outcast of the Islands*, underlie the later representations of feminism in *Chance*. While Gail Fraser analyzes *An Outcast of the Islands* as an almost propagandistic support for the Purity Campaign's political platform—to separate the races sexually and thereby "to keep the white descent 'pure' and the colonial authority 'efficient'" (124)—I maintain that the instability of this racial border—and the consequent impossibility of policing it—makes ambivalent the separation of the races, the regulation of racial identities, the purity of white descent, and the naturalized authority of white colonial rule, market supremacy, and patrimony in Conrad. With the bourgeois bedroom floating on the edge between the metropolis and the colony, female sexuality, in *Chance,* marks the instability of the identities through which colonial authority defines and sustains its powers.

Flora's sexuality is invoked through a symbolics of blackness, suggesting the dangers, to white reproduction, of white colonial settlement. In fact, as Sander Gilman has shown, representations of sexuality in women in the nineteenth and early twentieth centuries cited conventions of racial imagery, subtextually mixing bodily features from what empirical science would have claimed as different racial typologies. Questioning why the black servant (or nurse), so important for the figuration of ("white") female sexuality in Manet's 1862 painting *Olympia*, gets omitted in his 1877 portrait of the prostitute *Nana*, Gilman has traced a historical trajectory of women's sexuality as figuring the borders of white racial identity:

> Manet draws ... upon the vocabulary of signs associated by the late nineteenth century with the sexualized female.... Manet places her [Nana] in a position vis-à-vis the viewer ... which emphasizes the line of her buttocks, the steatopygia of the prostitute. Second, Nana is placed in such a way that the viewer ... can observe her ear. It is, to no one's surprise, Darwin's ear, a sign of the atavistic female. Thus we know where the black servant is hidden in *Nana.* She is hidden within Nana. For even her seeming beauty is but a sign of the black hidden within. All her external stigmata point to the pathology within the sexualized female. (1985: 102)

Gilman discusses a tradition of representation where shades of the Hottentot are still embedded in the figure of the sexualized ("white") female even when the black woman herself is removed from the background of the picture. Tracking the image of the Hottentot as a locus of both female sexuality (her sexual organs, her buttocks, her genitalia, and her labia majora are elongated, swelled, and overemphatic) and disease in the nineteenth century, Gilman notes, "What is most striking is that as she ages, the prostitute begins to appear more and more mannish. Billroth's *Handbook of Gynecological Diseases* links the Hottentot with the lesbian; here the link is between two other models of sexual deviancy, the prostitute and the lesbian. Both are seen as possessing physical signs that set them apart from the normal" (1985: 98). By pointing out the similarities, in Manet's painting and in Zola's novel that inspires it, between late-nineteenth century images of black women and images of sexualized ("white") women—their coterminous links to nature, to death, to disease, and to the voluptuousness of atavistic sexuality—Gilman argues that the sexualized female, the prostitute, in her tendencies toward lesbianism (as Zola's novel would warrant), is a cross-breed, but secretly so.

In *Chance,* the emergence of female sexuality is a factor through which the narrative is organized. The progressive configuring of sexuality in women is paralleled, in the text, to the story's passage toward the ends of empire. *Chance* moves from the de-eroticized setting of Fynes's home, where feminist politics is the mainstay of domestic life, to Flora's sexually charged entrance onboard a ship bound for the colonies. The generational split is, in fact, reflective of the histories of women in the changing political climate that feminism, at the time, was affecting. Before the turn of the nineteenth century, the New Woman was defined principally on the basis of her demands for access to the public sphere traditionally described, in late Victorian and early Edwardian social contexts, in male terms. According to Carroll Smith-Rosenberg (1989), first-generation New Women, who were in increasing numbers entering education and professional careers and, contingently, organizing all-women's living arrangements in college residences and settlement houses, did not significantly alter or challenge the discursive treatment of femininity as the embodiment of morality, respectability, and sexual purity. Their platform, Smith-Rosenberg argues, was much more aligned with an Enlightenment discourse on rights, individual autonomy, civic virtue, and self-determination.

In *Chance*, Mrs. Fyne, like the first-generation New Woman described by Smith-Rosenberg, defines feminism in terms of political issues, whereas Flora's femininity dangerously embraces sexuality. Mrs. Fyne's model of feminism based on political subjectivity and civic virtue was actually inadequate, Smith-Rosenberg continues, for the next generation of women who wanted the possibility of expressing themselves sexually. Appropriating the sexological rendition of the sexualized "mannish lesbian" from the writings of Havelock Ellis and Richard von Krafft-Ebing, these women repudiated purity, with its conceptualizations of female sexuality subordinated to political agency and tangential to men's active desire, reconfiguring an erotics of feminine desire as active and experimental. Signifying expressions of female sexuality such as Flora's, the "genital anomalies" and abnormal social conduct of the "woman on the make," moreover, were diagnosed within the medical literature as "sexually and racially dangerous" (271), manifesting the signs of atavism, racial contagion, moral breakdown, and evolutionary regression as physically and behaviorally recurrent. Allied with such medical models, nonconventional and financially solvent middle-class white women at the beginning of the twentieth century—successors to the first wave of feminism—inhabited an already existent figuration of sexuality in women as racially impure.

Reliant on the tradition of the literary imaging of the arguably desexualized New Woman in such novels as Henry James's *The Bostonians* (1886), *Chance* plays on these tensions in definitions of female sexuality. *The Bostonians* tells the story of Verena Tarrant's turning away from feminism and political activism, like Flora's rejection of Mrs. Fyne, through her progressive sexualization: she is increasingly seduced away from Olive's influence at the same time as she is increasingly sexualized as the willing object of desire under the gaze of the admiring Mr. Ransom. Feminism is depicted as contrary to sexual engagement. Like *Chance*, *The Bostonians* has elicited a barrage of criticism that, as Terry Castle has noted, raises questions about whether the intimacy between Olive Chancellor and Verena Tarrant is "really" a "lesbian love,"—"a feminine mystery," Ransom ruminates, "which must be allowed to take its course" (281). Against such social historians as Carroll Smith-Rosenberg and Lillian Faderman, who would position the beginnings of "lesbianism" at the early twentieth century, Castle argues that *The Bostonians*, following the tradition of representing intimacies between women since Marie Antoinette, gives "the *effect*, if not the actual reality, of a reciprocal lesbian desire" (165), a "ghostly" effect that is, Castle maintains, "nonexistent . . . [but] nonetheless *appears*" (46). This "effect," to which the criticism has responded, is created, according to Castle, in James' subtextual, intertextual, or "spectral" referencing of Emile Zola's 1880 novel *Nana,* with its allusions to the demimondaine and sexually explicit affair between Nana and Satin. Zola uses the alternatively violent, alternatively tender relationship between Nana and Satin, along with Nana's prostitution and her sexual manipulations of all classes of men, as the repository of an array of social vices (including gambling, horse-racing, adultery, theater, business speculation, and the unlimited, frivolous spending habits of the moneyed classes) and the apocalyptic sign of the Second Empire's imminent moral collapse. Flora—as Conrad inherits her from James, Zola, and the traditions on which they drew—is always on the verge of an illicit sexuality secretly evoked in her ever-narrowing proximity to the symptomology of atavism, a narrative of evolutionary regression literalized in her approach to the colonies.

Chance has a plot motivated to a certain degree by anxieties over Flora's fertility and the need of the narration to police and reinstate it. Flora needs to be rescued from the self-sufficiency, the noncompliance, with which Mrs. Fyne's emancipatory doctrine ensnares her, by marrying and reproducing. The relationship Flora has with Mrs. Fyne's feminism and with the governess's economic self-reliance is paralleled, in the text, with her obsessive insistence on caring for her father, thus linking the structural significance of a woman's independence to the economic closure of incest, her inaccessibility to sexual circulation and competitive male desire. Flora's development, then, depends on the retrieval of her ("white") femininity through Anthony's desire, consummated in his reproduction. The rescue theme follows, as Julie M. Johnson argues, the chivalric structures of quest adventures in Arthurian legend. The subtitles of the two sections of the novel, "Part I: The Damsel" and "Part II: The Knight," reflect a romantic ideal based on themes of rescue and possession:

> The "damsel," Flora de Barral, embodies the dual nature of Christian Grail—symbol and pagan fertility goddess—a conjunction which is characteristic of much quest literature in the Arthurian tradition. . . . We judge each character in light of the degree to which . . . he attempts to rescue her [Flora] from entrapment or to ensnare her further. . . . Through the connotations of this imagery she is linked to the fertility aspect of the Grail legends, and Marlow even refers to her at one point as a "vessel," making the relationship between sexuality and the Grail imagistically explicit. (221–22)

Though Johnson concludes that the ending, with the betrothal of Flora to Powell, conveys the success of the knights on their quest, the ambiguity of the ending is ultimately a distortion of romantic convention and suggests the incompleteness of Flora's rescue from pagan infertility into white motherhood. I explore here how Flora's "unnatural" unreproductiveness (of whiteness), and her sexualization through the gaze of the male knight-narrators, evoke symbolically the hidden internal presence of black femininity. "Miscegenation," Gilman adds, "embodies a fear not merely of interracial sexuality, but of its supposed result, the decline of population. For interracial marriages were seen as exactly parallel to prostitution in their barrenness" (1985: 107). The rescue of the vessel of the Grail in *Chance* is a desperate attempt to redeem the white man's reproduction by saving him from miscegenation.

Despite Anthony's infatuation with her, Flora made him promise that they would not, for the sake of her father, consummate their marriage, so that paternal authority works throughout the novel to defer Flora's reproductiveness. As an obstacle to the resolution that the novel seeks, de Barral is situated as a rival to Anthony. The obstacle preventing the conjugal consummation between Anthony and Flora is the incestuous circularity, the self-containment, of Flora's attentiveness to and preoccupation with her father. Like Almayer between Nina and Dain in *Almayer's Folly,* the Great de Barral is constantly standing in the way of Flora's engagement with Anthony, her turn toward a reproductive sexuality. "That man is getting tired of you," he tells her. "Let's get away" (383–84). Flora's idealization of and excessive devotion to her father obstructs a domestic resolution of her relationship with Anthony, exhibiting it, in its colonial situatedness, as an empty shell, a lifeless vessel. The suggestion that Flora will finally capitulate to Anthony's seductions works not only to compel the plot forward but also to question colonial policies of resettlement as an answer to the problem of concubinage. "If women were not a force of nature, blind in its strength and capricious in its power, they would not be mistrusted," Marlow reasons. "As it is one can't help it.... He [Anthony] had dealt with her masterfully. But man has captured electricity too. It lights him on his way, it warms his home, it will even cook his dinner for him—very much like a woman. But what sort of conquest would you call it?" (327). Flora's unreproductiveness reflects the threat that the colonial mission causes to domestic gender relations and hierarchies, the threat to economic control posed by insecure governance.

Flora's delayed marriage and later vow of sterility, for her own self-interest and her father's, mark her renunciation of her role in eugenic progress and racial survival, becoming, in a veiled way, a problem in the same way that feminism was seen as a problem. The "positive eugenics" discourse at the beginning of the twentieth century did construe motherhood, in opposition to feminism, as a woman's duty to her race, to civilization, and, therefore, to her gender. In his essay "eugenic feminist" (1911), C. W. Saleeby noted,

> It is that the best women, those favoured by Nature in physique and intelligence, in character and their emotional nature, the women who are increasingly to be found enlisted in the ranks of Feminism, and fighting the great fight for the Women's Cause, shall be convinced by the unchangeable and beneficial facts of biology, seen in the bodies and minds of women, and shall direct their efforts accordingly; so that they and those of their sisters who are of the same natural rank, instead of increasingly deserting the ranks of motherhood and leaving the blood of inferior women to constitute half of all future generations, shall on the contrary furnish an ever-increasing proportion of our wives and mothers, to the great gain of themselves, and of men, and of the future. (14)

Likewise, sexology tended to view the feminist "flight from motherhood" as a racial danger. William Lee Howard, in his 1900 article "Effeminate Men and Masculine Women," declares,

> The female possessed of masculine ideas of independence; the viragint who would sit in the public highways and lift up her pseudo-virile voice, proclaiming her sole right to decide questions of war or religion, or the value of celibacy and the curse of woman's impurity, and that disgusting antisocial being, the female sexual pervert, are simply different degrees of the same class—degenerates.... Should such a female be unfortunate enough to become a mother, she ceases to be merely amusing, and ... is then a menace to civilization, a producer of nonentities, the mother of mental and physical monstrosities who exist as a class of true degenerates until disgusted Nature, no longer tolerant of the woman who would be a man, or the man who would be a woman, allows them to shrink unto death. (687)

In much the same way as these women are anxiously scrutinized, becoming the objects around which the narratives of socio-medical discourse would develop, Flora's infertile marriage to Anthony is, in fact, obsessively watched and monitored by the textual movements and narrator-witnesses of *Chance*. Organizing the narrative structure of *Chance*, the excessive observations of Flora (as empty "vessel") by, among others, the crew members—and the anticipation the "vessel" produces textually—depict her, like the monstrously unmotherly and degenerate women featured in the scientific reports, as a disruption in the work world of men, a betrayal of the (colonial) civilizing mission, and therefore like a ship on the sea leading toward the colonial outpost, "uncertain," a "proverbial inconstancy," a "bewitching" (288).

As the discursive mobilization of motherhood was used to stigmatize femininities newly emerging through the women's movement, so a national elevation of motherhood as a "matter of Imperial importance," as Anna Davin has pointed out, was becoming a way of controlling and confining femininities. Mothers were made responsible, in scientific and public policy campaigns, for pervasive rises in infant mortality and the resulting perceived decrease in population that inhibited imperial expansion, settlement, and rule. "The maintenance of empire ...," cites Davin from J. L. Gavin, a prominent journalist, writing in 1905, "would be best based upon the power of a white population, proportionate in numbers, vigour and cohesion to the vast territories which the British democracies in the Mother Country and the Colonies control" (10).

Motherhood, instructed a 1909 article in *Eugenics Review* treating women's education, was an obligation "as much imperial as domestic and social, . . . [which would] arouse her to the imperative necessity of preparation, intelligent and sustained, for [its] fulfillment" (as cited in Davin, 22). Maternity insurance provisions were defended in a 1910 *Empire Review* article, alongside "lactation premiums," on the basis that they were "of greater vital importance to the race than old age pensions" (24). It was, according to Davin, maternal ignorance that was blamed for the decline in racial strength, population power, and British imperial dominance. Read through such contemporary discourses remaking motherhood as an imperial project, Flora's protracted celibacy and Anthony's subsequent "condition" (207)—his "betrayal," which distracts the crew—indicate a breakdown in the business, the labor, and the peopling of empire.

The suspense of the narrative depends on and revolves around anxieties aroused in watching the developments of Flora's ever-suspended sexual relations with the imperial captain Anthony and in speculating on the fate of the explosive "vessel" now only nominally in his charge. Textual tension is created as Flora's possibly incestuous desire, her sexual self-sufficiency—"the unusual in marital relations" (272)—adopted from Mrs. Fyne's feminism and the governess's inobsequiousness, obstructs her passage to motherhood—a successful resolution to Anthony's imperial governance and enterprise. The first mate Franklin, for instance, complains, "Did you ever hear of the captain's room being on the port side? Both of them stern cabins have been fitted up afresh like a blessed palace . . . , as if the Queen were coming with us. Of course the starboard cabin is the bedroom one, but the poor captain hangs out to port on a couch" (297). The pressure exerted on the narrative by Flora's continued barrenness is shadowed in the text by parallel uncertainties as to whether the ship will reach its destination in the colony and deliver its forty-ton cargo of dynamite. "Have you ever," asks Franklin, "seen a shipmaster walking his own deck as if he did not know what he had underfoot?" (302). What is underfoot that Anthony could not master was simultaneously both Flora and the dynamite being shipped to the colonies. The uncertainty in Anthony's mastery of the ship, of the colonial adventure with its stake in market growth and violence, is produced through the narrative's continually obstructed desire to know what is happening internally to Flora in that starboard bedroom below, to stabilize Flora as an object that the narrative can finally open up, see, and know. The ship's landing on the colony gets delayed as long as Flora's sexual development to motherhood.

Flora's "fate" (as Marlow calls it) exhibits that the maternal imperative of reproducing imperial subjects is, by definition, a hazardous project from the start: the potential of motherhood to reproduce whiteness in imperial subjects was coextensive with the threat that maternity itself was the place where colonial authority would lose coherence and explode. While motherhood was becoming a discursive site on which the limits of purity and racial identity were set, it was also already endangered with possibilities of contamination. Davin's analysis shows how the politics of mothering among the British middle classes maintained ideologies of racial health as controls for the economic and social organization of the working classes. Alternatively, motherhood was considered a place where racial impurities were inevitably entering undetected into the genetic stock. The anxious speculation on female sexualities—on whether in reproducing they would maintain the purity of their lineage—was coterminously evoking, for example, stories of animal husbandry in which females produced infertile hybrids and mongrels even when they were kept under strictest surveillance, discipline, domestic confinement, and control (Ritvo, 47). Flora's fertility is forestalled in her crossing of the imperial line.

By situating the story of *Chance* geographically in the sea between the metropolis and the colony and, conjunctively, by placing Flora in the passage from girlhood to adult sexuality, Conrad recreates the problem of female sexuality as an ambivalence and suspense that the colonial venture produces. The representation of femininity in *Chance* shows that, in Conrad, violations to the border regulating sexual relations in the colonies were producing themselves discursively inside narratives of femininity. Analyzing the lack of historical recounting of masters raping slaves in the United States, Abdul R. JanMohamed points out that secrecy and silence, as opposed to a Foucauldian-type discursive production, constitutes identities around the taboos of the racial-sexual border: "This deployment of silence, wherein those who could speak did not want to and those who did want to speak were prevented from doing so, produced racialized sexuality as a discursive formation. In this dynamic structure, where silence and repression play a strategic rather than a tactical or local role, sexuality becomes an even more dense transfer point for relations of power" (105). In its kinship with *Almayer's Folly* and *An Outcast of the Islands*, *Chance* demonstrates, however, that "racialized sexuality" was not exactly silent but instead written loudly through the discursive inscriptions of a troubled female sexuality.

But what is the real trouble with Almayer? What is his folly? In Conrad's novel, it is ambiguous whether the Arabs, or the final departure of his daughter Nina with her Malay prince, finally weakens the white man and impels him into an opium-induced fever of death. The Arabs, acquiring steam power, have taken over the river for their own commercial interests. Certainly, Arab trade advantage is a "savage intrusion" into Almayer's hopes of a prosperous commercialism, a deathly arrow flung into the enterprise, penetrating the white man's hopes of securing his home by securing market share. By destroying Almayer's ambitions for succeeding in business and trade, the ascendance of Arab capital and business venturism also inhibits his resolution of setting up a secure private arena, the domestic ideal.

In fact, the words "savage intrusion" in the text do not describe the Arabs' monopoly over new technologies, geographical spaces, and expanding markets. Instead, these words mark Almayer's anxiety over his betel-nut-chewing, witchlike, half-caste wife's continued influence over his daughter Nina: "One thing only disturbed his happiness; his wife came out of her seclusion, importing her green jacket, scant sarongs, shrill voice, and witch-like appearance, into his quiet life in the small bungalow. And his daughter seemed to accept that savage intrusion into her daily existence with wonderful equanimity" (37). Colonial competition is here treated as a domestic rupture where the conflict is narrated as a competitive struggle, between the parents on either side of a racial divide, for power over the daughter.

Almayer's Folly is Almayer's house. Built on the banks of the river, the house was to fulfill Almayer's dreams of splendor in civilization, transporting civilization into the interior of Malaysia. Establishing his betel-nut-chewing wife in the home that was to stand in for European civilization so desperately missed, Almayer, however, set up his ideal on insecure footing. For the wife did not respect the conventions of domestic femininity and sought its destruction through "outbursts of savage invective" (29), "burning the furniture, and tearing down the pretty curtains in her unreasoning hate of those signs of civilization" (29). Almayer maintains the illusion of solid domesticity, "stamp[ing] his foot to show the solidity of the neatly-fitting floors and expatiat[ing] upon the beauties and convenience of the building," for, he says, the foundation of a British national culture in Malaysia depended on the establishment of a discrete domestic sphere, the home, unalienated and impenetrable by market forces (39). The burning of the Folly, as Almayer himself collapses in opium dreams, illustrates the impossibility, the final destructibility of a (middle-class, "white") ideal femininity with its hereditary governance and paternal surveillance.

The wife's influence over Nina's identity interferes with Almayer's plans to set Nina up in a palace in Europe and integrate her completely in her white inheritance, to re-establish domestic space as under the father's control. During her time of education at Mrs. Vinck's in Singapore, Nina's criminal sexuality—sign of her mother's race—threatens to disrupt the ideal white feminine domestic, as her courtship with a banker attests. Nina's mother's stories still affect her physically, overtaking the moral rectitude in which her European education was supposed to train her. Hearing her mother's stories, Nina "saw with vague surprise the narrow mantle of civilised morality, in which good-meaning people had wrapped her young soul, fall away and leave her shivering and helpless as if on the edge of some deep and unknown abyss" (46). Nina's mixed-bloodedness make her susceptible to infringements of natural feminine virtue on which the domestic ideal would be sustained.

Nina's racial ambivalence, which is also an ambivalence of parental identification representing a color line—"a savage mother and a father walking about amongst pitfalls, with his head in the clouds, weak, irresolute, and unhappy" (46)—is internalized as the economic struggle for market ascendancy:

> Her young mind having been unskilfully permitted to glance at better things, and then thrown back again into the hopeless quagmire of barbarism, full of strong and uncontrolled passions, had lost the power to discriminate.... Whether they traded in brick godowns or on the muddy river bank ...,

> Nina saw only the same manifestations of love and hate and of sordid greed chasing the uncertain dollar in all its multifarious and vanishing shapes. (46–47)

Nina's identification with her mother is paralleled by the Arabs' gradual increase in claims on the river brought about by the mother's secret (sexual and/or economic) alliance with the fiercely competitive Arab traders. Directly before the British gave up to the Dutch their claims on the east side of the river, leaving the Arabs in control, Almayer's wife's almost incestuous meetings with the Rajah Lakamba open his house to malignant penetration. Almayer's domestic disruption brings about economic loss:

> Often on moonlight nights the belated fishermen of Sambir saw a small canoe shooting out from the narrow creek at the back of the white man's house, and the solitary occupant paddle cautiously down the river in the deep shadows of the bank; and those events, duly reported, were discussed round the evening fire far into the night with the cynicism of expressions common to aristocratic Malays. Almayer went on struggling desperately, but with a feebleness of purpose depriving him of all chance of success against men so unscrupulous and resolute as his rivals the Arabs. The trade fell away from the large godowns, and the godowns themselves rotted piecemeal. The old man's banker, Hudig of Macassar, failed, and with this went the whole available capital. (29)

Arab incursions simultaneously into white economic supremacy and white marriages are integrated closely and work to debilitate and exhaust Almayer's already enfeebled health and self-control, his masculinity, as he heads toward his final demise in opium disease.

This struggle over market share is played out on the body and in the racial blood of Nina as she comes of age: "For years she had stood between her mother and her father, the one so strong in her weakness, the other so weak where he could have been strong" (157). However, the "wonderful equanimity" with which Almayer believes Nina accepts her mother's Arab "intrusion" is perhaps not without its rifts and tensions. When Nina first sights Dain, her Malaysian prince, from behind a curtain, she struggles with her mother, vying for a better position from which to catch a more complete view of the newly arrived trader.

> Evidently Nina's strong curiosity was on the point of overcoming Mrs. Almayer's exalted sense of social proprieties. Hard breathing was distinctly audible, and the curtain shook during the contest, which was mainly physical, although Mrs. Almayer's voice was heard in angry remonstrance with its usual want of strictly logical reasoning, but with the well-known richness of invective.... "Veil your face, abandoned wretch! You white snake, I will not let you!" (57)

Nina is half of both races, here divided by a curtain. Her attraction to and curiosity about Dain the trader introduces her desire as aligned to a new economic order: she will pass, along with the white cultures and institutions of trade, away from her father and into the hands of a rising native elite. "You have come to the wrong house," Almayer responds to Dain's offer of alliance, "if you want to trade as you say" (56).

The replacement, which Nina's pretensions of marriage to Dain represent, of European mercantilism by Malaysian governance, discloses a situation reminiscent of Homi Bhabha's colonial mimesis—"the difference between being English and being Anglicized" (1987: 322)—where the colonized subject is reformed, constructed around a difference that is recognizable but still "Other," a difference that is the same *"but not quite"* (318; original emphasis). Bhabha claims that the repeatability of colonial identities belies any naturalization of colonial power by proving it imitable, "the final irony of partial representation" (321), but he does not include the role gender might play in this mimetic process. Dain's appropriation of Almayer's position and inheritance, through his marriage to Nina, entails a partial substitution that, as Bhabha says, makes a mockery of power by imitating it with a difference, by diffusing it, recreating it as "Other."

Dain's Malaysia will repeat, the text suggests, the "'normalized' knowledges and disciplinary powers" (318) of Almayer's colonial forms of ownership, paternalism, control, and alliance, and yet repeat them with a difference. Nina's central position as an object in this power negotiation projects gender and femininity in particular as the site in Conrad's text where racial differences are negotiated and racial identities created, imitated, and disrupted. In *Almayer's Folly*, colonial presence undermines itself by de-essentializing and denaturalizing its own authority, that is, by showing the representation and reproduction of its own identity, as Bhabha says, in native difference. Almayer's colonial desire, to repeat white identity and its presence through the establishment of European-style homes in Malay, is suspended when it is instigated through Almayer's wife's otherness, her not-quite-white femininity: "You are my daughter now," she tells Nina. "Never shall you go back to that house" (155).

Nina's gender identifications are intertwined thematically with the ways in which the borders of racial identities and colonial powers are constituted and deployed, done and undone in the text. When Nina identifies with her mother, with the nonwhite, she appears physically as racial difference exhibited through sexuality and desire, a partial resemblance, something not quite feminine, but almost:

> The squareness of lower jaw, the full red lips, the mobile nostrils, and the proud carriage of the head gave the impression of a being half-savage, untamed, perhaps cruel, and corrected the liquid softness of the almost feminine eye, that general characteristic of the race ... [Nina] felt a hitherto unknown feeling of shyness, mixed with alarm and some delight, enter and penetrate her whole being. Confused by those unusual sensations she stopped in the doorway and drew the lower part of the curtain across her face, leaving only half a rounded cheek, a stray tress, and one eye exposed, wherewith to contemplate the gorgeous and bold being. (59)

Hybridity implies no point of intersection or amalgamation here between the races but a radical ontological and economic segregation instead, a colonial divide—a curtain—located between unmixable biological differences, savagery and intrusion on one side, in the desire expressed in the returned gaze, and modesty on the other. In *Almayer's Folly,* Nina's sexualization makes her, as Homi Bhabha put it, "almost the same, but not white" (322; original emphasis).

Nina's whiteness is always in doubt, even by Almayer himself. Almayer's incomprehension of her identity, his projection of her as radically Other, leads him incessantly to observe her, watch her features, scrutinize the details of her physique, just as Flora in *Chance* is observed by the narrators. Nina's racial otherness becomes an object of Almayer's and the text's desire for access and mastery.

> As he [Almayer] lay looking ardently in her face, watching her tears, her parted lips, her very breath, he was uneasily conscious of something in her he could not understand.... He felt something invisible that stood between

> them, something that would let him approach her so far, but no farther. No desire, no longing, no effort of will or length of life could destroy this vague feeling of their difference. . . . She was his, and yet she was like a woman from another world. (194)

Almayer's interest, his ambivalence, focuses on Nina's racial features, which become Othered through his gaze, his ardor, and his longing. Her racial difference represents the material difference through which desire operates in the text.

The rivalry between Nina and her mother for the view of Dain is repeated later in the novel between Nina and a native woman, the Siamese slave girl Taminah. Taminah is triply enslaved: the last wife of the Malaysian Bulangi, she frequently comes under violent attack by his numerous other wives. Almost a spirit, a "vague shape," or "the shadow of a driving cloud" (162) in her ability to appear and disappear without notice, Taminah, like Nina's mother, incarnates the passion of the island: mean and vengeful, she threatens to obstruct the romance, the pairing of Nina and Dain in marriage. It is Taminah, in the end, who awakens Almayer to the lovers' plot and, in cryptic sentences that resist comprehension and mastery, incites him to try to stop their departure. "The figure of a woman standing in the steely light, her hands stretched forth in a suppliant gesture, . . . the obstinate phantom floated the murmur of words that fell on his ears in a jumble of torturing sentences, the meaning of which escaped the utmost efforts of his brain" (165).

Taminah is jealous. She is in love with Dain. She sees Nina as a hindrance to her own desire. But Taminah's incessant watch over Nina serves, within the text, to reinforce Nina's position as an object that needs constantly to be watched, reinforcing the erotic objectification that has marked, throughout the novel, Nina's changing racial identifications:

> She wanted to cry out; to rush at them and tear their vague shadows apart; to throw Nina into the smooth water, cling to her close, hold her to the bottom where that man could not find her. . . . She should have liked Dain to be dead, so as to be parted from that woman—from all women. She felt a strong desire to see Nina, but without any clear object. She hated her, and feared her, and she felt an irresistible impulse pushing her towards Almayer's house to see the white woman's face, to look close at those eyes, to hear again that voice. (122)

Taminah's presence threatens to prevent the union, constantly creating obstacles to defer or inhibit the meetings between Dain and Nina and their eventual plans to elope. Delaying the projected union between colonial governance and the rise of native trade, Taminah's violent, even criminal desire to see Nina plays the role, in the text, of creating suspense, blocking the colonial alliance from reproducing itself.

Conrad explains Taminah's obsession with obstructing Nina and Dain's courtship as narcissistic egoism. Taminah's watch over Nina is prefigured, before the sighting of the canoe, in her contemplation of her self: "And when the sun was near its setting she walked to the bathing-place and heard it as she stood on the tender grass of the low bank, her robe at her feet, and looked at the reflection of her figure on the glass-like surface of the creek" (119). This silent absorption in the face of her own naked image reflected, is interrupted, cut through with pain and anger by the drifting-in of Nina's "long canoe . . . bearing the two lovers into the white mist of the great river" (120). By looking at herself, Taminah creates an air of expectancy, suspense, and desire around Nina's entrance.

The construction of Dain's desire for Nina reproduces images of Taminah's violent watch over Nina. In Dain's eyes, in his projected fantasy, Nina becomes the savage, violent passion, that characterized her, previously, in Taminah's narcissistic identification. In other words, Dain imagines Nina's sexualization as the passion of the island:

> She drew back her head and fastened her eyes on his in one of those long looks that are a woman's most terrible weapon; a look that is more stirring than the closest touch, and more dangerous than the thrust of a dagger, because it also whips the soul out of the body, but leaves the body alive and helpless, to be swayed here and there by the capricious tempests of passion and desire; a look that enwraps the whole body, and that penetrates into the innermost recesses of the being, bringing terrible defeat in the delirious uplifting of accomplished conquest. (177)

Dain's fantasy of Nina projects eroticism as the "general characteristic of her race," that "liquid softness in her almost-feminine eye." As Nina's image is constructed through Dain's fantasy and Taminah's anger, her eroticization seems to draw on the same sets of physical features and terrible incomprehensibility—the fear of the eye looking back—as were remarked in Almayer's former exclamations over her racial difference. Nina's sexuality reveals the ambivalences of colonial power, the place where it is both authorized and undermined. The narrative of desire circulating around Nina suggests the instability of colonial rule and paternal authority, its heritage of purity. As barbaric aggressor and conqueror, Nina, in Dain's dream, threatens civilization and masculinity with "terrible defeat." She portends Almayer's financial ruin and domestic devastation as the Arabs, usurping the signs of colonial immanence—home, family, property, and rationality—make a parody of his capital conquest.

Nina's difference from the domestic ideal, which would establish, by repeating, European culture in Malay, "rearticulates," as Homi Bhabha says, "[colonial] presence in terms of its 'otherness,' that which it disavows" (324). The "path you [Almayer] would have wished me to follow," Nina says when she is, after Almayer's discovery and to his consternation, about to depart with Dain, "has been closed to me by no fault of my own" (196–97). In *Almayer's Folly,* colonial difference is represented as the ever-suspended ideal of domestic femininity through which colonial authority is constituted. Nina's flight from her father's home, from his Folly, underscores the confusion of colonial power's legitimization, the certainty of patrimony, of heredity (both racial and economic). The insecurity of whiteness, of colonial presence, is treated as the insecurity of an insular white femininity, Almayer's failed legacy: "That," he thinks, "was his idea of his duty to himself—to his race—to his respectable connections; to the whole universe unsettled and shaken by this frightful catastrophe of his life" (199).

Conrad's next novel, *An Outcast of the Islands,* further explores how femininity became a problem when colonial governance and market control lost their credibility and ideological domination. When Aïssa first appears, she is almost indiscernible from the thickets of trees that surround her, the primal forest; she is "a vision of blackness darker than the deepest shade of the forest" (68). Fusing with the forest, she hypnotizes and overwhelms the white man who watches as if "an invisible force made up of surprise and curiosity and desire spun him round" leaving him with "a sense of irreparable loss" (69), "a sense of immense sadness as after some great and irreparable loss" (73). To her, the white man, Willems, coming into the forest where white men never go, is "of the victorious race. . . . He appeared to her with all the fascination of a great and dangerous thing; of a terror vanquished, surmounted, made a plaything of" (75). As they have sex on the forest floor near the river, Willems capitulates to the force of the forest in her, beholding the terror, seeing himself empty of the power of being white and masculine:

> But in the sudden darkness of her going he would be left weak and helpless, as though despoiled violently of all that was himself. He who had lived all his life with no preoccupation but that of his own career, contemptuously indifferent to all feminine influence, full of scorn for men that would submit to it, if ever so little; he, so strong, so superior even in his errors, realized at last that his very individuality was snatched from within himself by the hand of a woman. Where was the assurance and pride of his cleverness; the belief in success, the anger of failure, the wish to retrieve his fortune, the certitude of his ability to accomplish it yet? Gone. All gone. All that had been a man within him was gone. (77)

In this first series of encounters, Willems's racial identity, his whiteness, is irreparably expressed through his sexual identity, his masculinity proven through conquest as proof of competitive superiority: "He was indeed a man! ... of the victorious race" (75). Aïssa, in all the primalness of the forest she embodies, makes a plaything of his whiteness and his civility that make him a man. Conrad's depiction of the complexities of colonial power is written through the "marginal vision of castration" (318)—of repetition and difference—that Homi Bhabha places at the center of colonial discourse. Yet Conrad, in dramatizing Aïssa and Willems's embattled attractions, indicates the gender trouble that such colonial fetishization of difference orchestrates, a point that Bhabha, in his focus on the institutional regulation of racial identities, elides. In ironizing Willems's assurance and pride and ambition, Aïssa, "with the unerring intuition of a primitive woman confronted by a simple impulse" (75), sees him "ready to be enslaved" (75). Aïssa's threat of possessing him, of appropriating and menacing his self-command, going "beyond the subject's lack of priority (castration) to a historical crisis in the conceptuality of colonial man" (Bhabha, 1987: 323), poses gender difference as a racial defense.

The connection between Aïssa and ecology has been taken by feminist critic Ruth Nadelhaft to mean that Conrad was aware and critical of colonial industrialism's ravaging of nature. To Nadelhaft, Aïssa represents nature's refuge: "This analysis establishes immediately the connection between a political awareness of the cost of Western culture and the ecological cost, the cost to female power and its integration into a pre-industrial way of life" (1991: 10). The retributive role that Aïssa plays here, however, is not simply nature's and woman's resistance to an encroaching power that would rout it. Aïssa is neither heroicized nor particularly concerned with conservation; in the end, she is unsuccessful, transformed into an aged and miserable witch. Like Nadelhaft, I do not propose that Aïssa is therefore just another instance of the "castrating" or "phallic mother," as psychoanalytic critics such as Bernard C. Meyer have claimed, nor, following Torgovnick's reduction, that Conrad's native women exemplify the simple collapse of "the feminine" into "the primitive." Aïssa's relation to nature, in fact, destabilizes her femininity—"the crash," Willems thinks, "of his own falling house"—by providing her with a subjective desire that is not quite feminine and threatens him with her imminent conquest over his masculinity where the supremacy of his race resides. "And he looked at her," Conrad narrates,

> standing above him, her head lost in the shadow of broad and graceful leaves that touched her cheek; while the slender spikes of pale green orchids streamed down from amongst the boughs and mingled with the black hair that framed her face, as if all those plants claimed her for their own—the animated and brilliant flower of all that exuberant life which, born in gloom, struggles for ever towards the sunshine. Every day she came a little nearer. (76)

Aïssa's imitation of colonial presence, her repeating its control and possession, depends on the exuberance of a nature beyond the pall, personified through the lack of regulation of its desire, its undomesticability. The ecological aspect, if one can be talked about in relation to Conrad at all, does not then represent femininity's revenge, nor femininity's flight into a preindustrial realm of plenitude, but instead an expression of gender ambivalence through a narrative of power appropriation, desire, and disruption on a racial border, and the resulting need for dominance.

Aïssa's sexual advances turn Willems into "a masquerading specter of the once so very confidential clerk of the richest merchant in the islands," dirty, looking "like some ascetic dweller in a wilderness" (92), with "long, tangled hair" (87), and with eyes "which glittered deep down in the sockets like the last sparks amongst the black embers of a burnt-out fire" (88). In effect, Willems "goes native," "producing a partial vision of the colonizer's presence" (Bhabha, 1987: 321). Her passion empties him of identity, presence, and power. In their scene of reunion after the Arabs have separated them in order to blackmail Willems for their commercial advantage, he experiences her excessive sensuality as an "irreparable loss," as impotency and irrationality:

> With that look she drew the man's soul away from him through his immobile pupils, and from Willems' features the spark of reason vanished under her gaze and was replaced by an appearance of physical well-being, an ecstasy of the senses which had taken possession of his rigid body; an ecstacy that drove out regrets, hesitation and doubt, and proclaimed its terrible work by an appalling aspect of idiotic beatitude. He never stirred a limb, hardly breathed, but stood in stiff immobility, absorbing the delight of her close contact by every pore. (140)

His "expression of being taken possession of" (141) makes him aware that he is a potential victim of her violence and conquest, that his standing as authority within such colonial relations could be reversed as somebody else took possession of him. When her blind father, "kneeling above him, [holding] the kriss in his hand" (149), tries to stab him in the dark after love-making, "she sat motionless as if she had been part of the sleeping earth, then suddenly he saw her big sombre eyes open out wide in a piercing stare and felt the convulsive pressure of her hands pinning his arms along his body" (149). Coming to the realization that, given over to "the unknown things, . . . those motives, impulses, desires he had ignored," he is defenseless against the violence, Willems sees Aïssa as the one who, extracting from him his male identity in the white and rational world, would make his body lifeless, an empty authority, devitalized by her abundant passion and sensuality: "He was in the grip of horrible fear, of a fear whose cold hand robs its victim of all will and of all power; of all wish to escape, to resist, or to move; which destroys hope and despair alike, and holds the empty useless carcass as if in a vise under the coming stroke" (149).

The violence of the daggerlike thrust in her not-quite-feminine eye creates Aïssa as a sign of racial and gender difference. As Aïssa herself specifies, she is uneasy with the name, the sign "woman" because of the difference, the violence, sometimes in her blood, sometimes in the colonial history of her people:

> I am a woman! Your eyes see that, . . . but can you see my life? I also have heard—. . . I also have heard the voice of fire-arms; I also have felt the rain of young twigs and of leaves cut up by bullets fall down about my head; I also know how to look in silence at angry faces and at strong hands raised high grasping sharp steel. I also saw men fall dead around me without a cry of fear and of mourning; and I have watched the sleep of weary fugitives, and looked at night shadows full of menace and death with eyes that knew nothing but watchfulness. And . . . I have faced the heartless sea, held on my lap the heads of those who died raving from thirst, and from their cold hands took the paddle and worked so that those with me did not know that one man more was dead. (245)

In a sense, Aïssa has usurped the terms of colonial authority by turning back the violent gaze by which colonial power conferred meanings and assigned identities to those on the other side of the color line.

The struggle, in the end, between Aïssa and Willems over the possession of Willems's revolver, images Willems as "a man awakened by the crash of his own falling house" (77), a man whose racial supremacy is challenged through the destabilizing of his masculinity, which is the basis of his economic, political, and domestic solvency. He meditates obsessively that he cannot leave the island without his revolver and "made up his mind quickly for a rush to the house, to grab his revolver and . . .—a vision of things done swiftly with enraged haste—to save his prestige, his superiority—something of immense importance" (352). He cannot, he seems to think, return to his position as a man in the white world without firearms. Then, Aïssa appears holding his revolver.

> He dared not go unarmed. He made a long stride, and saw her raise the revolver. He noticed that she had not cocked it, and said to himself that, even if she did fire, she would surely miss. Go too high; it was a stiff trigger. He made a step nearer—saw the long barrel moving unsteadily at the end of her extended arm. He thought: This is my time. . . . He bent his knees slightly, throwing his body forward, and took off with a long bound for a tearing rush. He saw a burst of red flame before his eyes, and was deafened by a report that seemed to him louder than a clap of thunder. Something stopped him short, and he stood aspiring in his nostrils the acrid smell of the blue smoke that drifted from before his eyes like an immense cloud. . . . And he

> saw her very far off, throwing her arms up, while the revolver, very small, lay on the ground between them (360).

Willems's inability to grab the revolver and make his escape, in this scene so inundated with sexual allusions, insinuates that what is at stake in the colonial engagement between the races is the "irreparable loss" of an access to instrumental violence, "his prestige" and "superiority."

The struggle over the revolver is foreshadowed by another struggle immediately preceding this scene of Willems's death: his wife suddenly and unexpectedly appears on the island to take Willems home. The two women become embroiled in a scuffle over whether Willems will proceed back to the island or away across the river.

> She [Aïssa] stared at Joanna [Willems' wife], while between the short gusts of broken laughter she raved.... The long hair, released, fell scattered over her shoulders, framing in its blackness the wild exaltation of her face. "Drive her off, Peter. Drive off the heathen savage," persisted Joanna.... "Look," cried Aïssa. "Look at the mother of your son! She is afraid. Why does she not go from before my face? Look at her. She is ugly." ... As Aïssa stepped back again nearer to the tree, [Joanna] let go her husband's arm, rushed at her madly, slapped her face, then, swerving round, darted at the child who, unnoticed, had been wailing for some time, and, snatching him up, flew down to the waterside, sending shriek after shriek in an access *[sic]* of insane terror. (358–59)

This "wild exaltation" and violent passion seem to escalate, this time, over reproduction. When Willems commands Joanna, "Snatch the boy—and my revolver there" (358), the means to violence and reproduction are linked as the two things that must be saved and brought away into civilization, staving off the difference, the "irreparable loss" and restoring the lost powers of civilization. The difference between the two women is configured in Aïssa's now emphatic awareness of her infertility. Aïssa's womanhood is clearly differentiated from the legitimate femininity of Joanna, who is capable of bearing ("white") sons. "To her!" screams Aïssa. "To her—the mother of him who will speak of your wisdom, of your courage. All to her. I have nothing. Nothing. Take, take" (358). Though dead, Willems at last conquers, having assured and saved his line of "white" descent and authority in masculinity.

The appearance of Joanna on the island not only brands Aïssa as a woman almost but not quite feminine because she is incapable of giving birth. Also, her appearance on the island discloses that Aïssa is triply enslaved, as she says, "the slave of a slave" (358), as Willems's second wife. But the scene is also reminiscent of the prior scene, discussed earlier, where Willems appears "gone native" with "long, tangled hair" (87). For Willems's transformation, brought about in his sex act with Aïssa, threatens to awaken the white child Nina, whom her father, Almayer, seeks to protect. The possibility that Willems would disturb the child is linked by Almayer to the possibility that the child's awakening would in turn disrupt the sanctity of civilization in the white man's home: "Don't shout like this. Do you think yourself in the forest with your . . . your friends? This is a civilized man's house. A white man's. Understand?" (88). Soliciting a loan from Almayer for the purpose of setting up his own home, where "I could have her all to myself . . .—under my own influence—to fashion—to mould—to adore—to soften—to" (92), Willems intrudes into civilization, represented by the sleeping child, in order to naturalize through domestication his relationship with Aïssa: "'After all it's natural,' went on Willems, without paying any attention to Almayer—'it's natural that she would expect the advantages which . . .'" (92). Almayer denies any aid, leading to Willems's desperate backing of the Arabs' insidious plan to win the river for their own commercial mastery. The impossibility of domesticating Aïssa in a home with a sleeping white child parallels and even incites the unnatural rise in Arab enterprise, industrialization, and trade advantage.

The aggressive negotiation between the two men over the body of the sleeping child finally arouses Nina who, repeating the words of her white father—"Pig! Pig! Pig!"—drives Willems away (94). The white child represents a defense against the intrusion of the voices of the forest, which would open the domestic to Arab economic ascendancy and the de-authentication, through native appropriations and hybrid reproductions, of colonial authority. Says Almayer, "What is the meaning of your veiled threats? . . . The Arabs have been hanging about outside the river for years—and I am still the only trader here; the master here. Do you bring me a declaration of war?" (93). Because she and Willems are prohibited from building a home together by the repudiation of the white child, Aïssa becomes, in essence, the figure of racial difference, almost but not quite feminine. It is not clear, then, that the native women "resort to cunning and subversion to destroy the identity of the very white men who enslave them" (1986: 151) and succeed in "limiting the effect of white power . . . revealing the liberating potential of native vitality, and . . . projecting the doom of male European colonialism" (152), as Ruth Nadelhaft argues. Instead, native women, by mocking the domestic ideal of civilization, represent the limit-case through which colonial authority draws, vitalizes, reinstates, *and* disavows its difference.

In both novels, Conrad evinces how interracial sexual relations work to undermine, to alter while reconfirming, the configurations of the politics of reproduction and the colonial legacy, the institution of patrimony, they would engender. In fact, at the time Conrad was writing, miscegenation and the politics of sex in the colonies were being renegotiated both legislatively and logistically. Legal and social prohibitions on interracial sex, by emphasizing anxieties over prostitution, concubinage, chastity, cleanliness, and health, were complicit in foregrounding fears about barrenness elicited in the very terms of purity discourse. Responding to the British Purity Campaign's lobbying for legal restrictions on prostitution and white slavery, in 1909 the Houses of Parliament passed the Crewe Circular, entitled "Immoral Relations with Native Women," which was to curtail access to concubinage, on threats of dismissal, among the newcoming colonial officers in some specified colonies (including Malay). The circular warned each new recruit of the "'disgrace and official ruin which will certainly follow' should he enter into 'arrangements of concubinage with girls or women belonging to the native populations,'" as such relations "'will seriously impair his capacity for useful work in the Service in which it is his duty to set an honorable example to all with whom he comes in contact'" (as cited in Hyam, 157). According to Ronald Hyam, the reorganization of interracial sexual relations in the colonies, spurred by the Purity Campaign's struggle against prostitution and sexually transmittable diseases, was part of a larger campaign to refashion the concept of masculinity: "By 1914 the whole British concept of masculinity—not least in the public schools—had been redefined, partly in the name of empire, to mean not sexual prowess and maturity but sexual restraint and 'cleanliness'" (71). Hyam goes on to note that "the more general presence of white women in colonial communities" (209), as wives relocated in the colonies, was a more forceful encouragement to restricting sex between the races. *Chance* stages the passage of white women to the colonies and the enjoining possibility of interracial reproduction.

However, Conrad indicates that the movement of white women into colonial spaces did not so much help to consolidate a racial border but instead intensified the apprehension surrounding the positioning of femininity as the guardian and defense of white racial authority. In fact, as Ann Laura Stoler (1991) has argued, concubinage in the colonies, though a beneficial arrangement in the nineteenth century for labor control, permanent settlement, cultural adaptation, salary curtailment, and the provision of domestic service for civil servants, later was a dangerous incursion criticized on moral grounds. The resultant imperialist impulse to regulate racial purity through the importation of white wives was not actually executed all at once and across the board but instead underwent various degrees of implementation depending on logistical and residential provisions, rank, perceived dangers in particular locales, and the embeddedness of the interracial domestic institution of concubinage in a particular colonial setting. Though the presence of white women in the colonies did lead to changing arrangements, refining settlements, and identifying mannerisms, "maintaining the social rituals of racial difference" (1991: 65), partitioning residential compounds, and marking the borders of racial-cultural activities and social spaces, colonial white women were also surrounded by a barrage of discursive concern over racial infractions: reports of rape and of perceived transgressions of colonials into white private spaces circulated preponderantly.

In addition, the drawing of racial differences through restricting the sexualities of white women in the colonies was undermined by the coterminous questioning of whether white femininity could hold itself, physically and morally, in custody of the ideal, the exemplary essence of pure whiteness, civilization, and morality.[5] "The Indies mixed marriage law of 1898," Stoler cites as an example, "relegated those European women to native status who chose cohabitation over marriage and chose native men over the European-born on the argument that if these women were really European they would never have made such inappropriate choices" (1995: 183). "Light literature" and the pornographic aesthetics of scientific investigations joined to produce racial taxonomies within and around the troubles that femininities posed for colonial bureaucratic control.[6] "In Dutch colonial novels" and colonial "gynecological stud[ies]" (184), for example, "women of European status but of Indies birth, or of mixed-blood and common class origin appear as sensual, erotically charged beings, driven by passion in ways that "pure-blood" middle-class European women void and supposedly bereft of desire were not" (183).

A text by J. Allen Gilbert (1920) exemplifies the way in which the feminist New Woman invert secretly adopts the medical heritage of the construction of race to which I am referring. Dr. Gilbert does a physical examination of his patient "H.," the "homo-sexual" in need of treatment, and finds that "the hips, while relatively larger than would conform to the strictly male type, still fell short of the average female contour. The breasts, when in standing position, presented nothing to suggest deviation from the female type, except, possibly, an unusual flabbiness. . . . The clitoris was abnormally large" (320). Tracing the history of the stereotype of the Hottentot, female desire, and pathological sexuality through the nineteenth century, Gilman cites sources that describe her as having such abnormal features as a "'Hottentot apron,' a hypertropy of the labia and nymphae" (as observed by François Levaillant and John Barrow, travelers to Africa, and published in 1901) (85), "a bottom out of all proportion" (from a British novel, 1899) (91), and flabby breasts (from Saint-Hilaire and Frédéric Cuvier's *Histoire naturelle des mammifères avec des figures originales* (1824) (1985: 86). Gilbert's depiction of his standard invert borrows its characteristics from a standard repertoire of biological features already associated with the physiognomy of the black female. A 1867 dissection report of a bushwoman, for instance, observes that she has a thickness of fat in her buttocks (190). Proceeding right along, the scientists measure her "Generative Organs" assiduously, recording lengths, shapes, and distances between the parts, to conclude that "Mammae flaccid and elongated" (208), "3″ in diameter at the base, and about the same from base to apex" (196), the "glans clitoridis . . . each side 2″ long" (207), and "the remarkable development of the labia minora, or nymphae, which is so general a characteristic of the Hottentot and Bushman race, was sufficiently well marked to distinguish these parts at once from those of any of the ordinary varieties of the human species" (208). Gilbert's solution to the "problem" of H.'s "inconvenient" "condition of abnormal inversion" is to "adopt the procedure," upon H.'s own demand (he says), of sterilization, oöphorectomy, and hysterectomy (321).

Certainly, Flora, like H., because of her barrenness—her suspended motherhood on the colonial divide—is an object of constant surveillance, as both the primary knight-narrators (Marlow, Powell, and Marlow's unnamed companion) and the secondary characters (principally the Fynes, the governess, her father de Barral, and the men on the ship) are consistently vying for a position from which to view her. So it is ironic, perhaps, the discomfort that such characters feel when Flora turns back the stare, creating emotional dissonance in the power that the others have been able to exercise over her: "Moreover, she [Mrs. Fyne] had caught the girl looking at her in a peculiar way at times. Oh no!—it was not an evil look—it was an unusual expression which one could not understand. And when one remembered that her father was in prison, shut up together with a lot of criminals and so on—it made one uncomfortable. . . . And that was somewhat perverse—wasn't it?" (179–80). The turning back of the stare reminds Mrs. Fyne of Flora's hereditary past, where her father had criminally wedged his way into the business establishment and its society by claiming the signs of middle-class status. In a certain way, Flora's father exposed the arbitrariness of the middle class by showing how its privileges and prestige can almost be easily and convincingly worn by another.

Though Flora's figure is excessively white and female, "appealing . . . and . . . desirable" (201), with smooth white skin, seemingly blue eyes (423), slight hips, and a fine, pointed chin, and though she dresses in the same flowing skirts which H. wore "as a trademark of femininity" to shield her difference from the social gaze, her stare itself demonstrates the possibility of racial difference. As Sander Gilman points out, it is often the gaze, "the vivacity of the eye" (44), "eyelid retraction, and a compulsive stare" (148), which evoke the regressive disposition of disease—the mark of difference, a sign of beleaguered heredity and its diseases, adds Gilman, including sterility. In fact, there is a constant referencing in the novel to the idea of Flora's eye color as something that, even with everybody watching her, nobody knows for sure. "You don't know the colour of her eyes," Marlow screams at Mr. Fyne when they are discussing how Flora seduced Anthony by making "desperate eyes" at him (243). "You do talk to that white-faced, black-eyed," winces first-mate Franklin to the young Powell. And Powell responds "in a disdainful tone that Mrs. Anthony's eyes were not black." "I wish to God," Franklin rejoins, "she had never set them on the captain, whatever colour they are" (304). Marlow remarks upon Flora's "darkening eyes" and "fixed stare" (199), which the text, via Marlow, fervently watches. Flora's eyes seem to be a particularly ambivalent site for determining her identity and a source of her power.

The narrative's inability to focus on Flora as its referent means that the text is always anxiously moving toward a place where she can be discovered and observed but a place from which she is never quite visible. During Marlow's first significant meeting with Flora, Flora is standing on the edge of a precipice about to take, he will learn, a suicidal leap. Later, when Fyne and Marlow are searching for her (for she had run off, it is later said, to London, with Anthony, who would become at least nominally her husband), they enter the quarry below: "These bushes were heavy with dew. There were also concealed mudholes in there. We crept and tumbled and felt about with our hands along the ground. We got wet, scratched, and plastered with mire all over our nether garments. Fyne fell suddenly into a strange cavity—probably a disused lime-kiln" (53). The obsessive policing that the characters, through gazing, perform on Flora's body, is interspersed by the moments, like this one, when she disappears, "a transient, phantom-like girl" (50) (like Taminah); the text then commences a restless and desperate search for her whereabouts. As Marlow and Fyne descend searching into dark passages of earth and moisture, the scene becomes uncannily similar to the one in which the heroes of Rider Haggard's 1887 novel *She*, a work that much influenced Conrad, travel into the "very womb of the Earth" to find, in Africa, the key to immortality in the possession and knowledge of a land immersed in black feminine traits: "The slope was very steep, and often precipitous, but it was nowhere impassable.... [We] discovered that, like the first long passage down which we had passed through the cliff before we reached the quivering spur, it had to all appearance been torn in the bowels of the rock by the terrific force of some explosive gas" (286).[7] The quarry into which Flora is about to "fall" when Marlow finds her and rescues her but from which, in this instance, she is hauntingly (never really convincingly) missing, reflects the features of the oversexualized female body, the blackness, the wide hips, the overpowerful and excessive excretions of a nature overgrown, consuming, possessive, and violently aggressive.

The never-resolved possibility that Flora might have actually fallen connects her, through identification, to her father. Having been imprisoned for his criminal enterprise, he seemed as though he "had been down to the Nether Region" (347). Just as Almayer's face resembled "the blank wall of a prison enclosing sin, regrets, and wasted life, in the cold indifference of mortar and stones" (196) after Nina left him, de Barral carries with him "the appalling tainted atmosphere of its [the prison's] silent abode" (245). Identification with the father through the fall is, according to Diana Fuss, a standard image for what will later—after Freud—be recognized as lesbian representation, signifying "a gravitational fall back into preoedipality" and often represented through a lady who has "fallen" in social position, having to earn her own living and thus not assuming the proper role of domestic ("middle class") femininity. Not only does the homosexual patient desire to "rescue" her lady love-object from her base economic circumstances in which she has fallen, Freud argues in his 1920 case "Psychogenesis of a Case of Homosexuality in a Woman"; also, the patient's suicidal fall represents, for Freud, her fantasy of becoming a "fallen woman" through bearing the father's child.

In *Chance,* the gender trouble and cross-gender identifications that Freud remarks is played out as a narrative of the colonial border. The Victorian reinvention of paternal authority as the referent around which gender difference is thought occurs simultaneously, McClintock observes, "when the emergence of the imperial bureaucracy was depriving the image of the father of symbolic power as the designated symbol of paternal power" (92). In McClintock's account, the Victorian governess represented problems in the new class structure that was calling into question paternal power. *Chance* is the tale of a white woman's passage to the colonies in which Conrad explores some of the problems inherent in the metropolitan class structures back home. Induced by her father's conviction for fraudulent business practices, Flora's "fall" parallels the fate of the governess, who took charge of Flora's upbringing after her mother's death. "Of course," interjects Marlow,

> all the chances were that de Barral should have fallen upon a perfectly harmless, naïve, usual, inefficient specimen of respectable governess for his daughter; or on a commonplace silly adventuress who would have tried, say, to marry him or work some other sort of common mischief in a small way. Or again he might have chanced on a model of all the virtues, or the repository of all knowledge, or anything equally harmless, conventional, and middle class. All calculations were in his favour; but, chance being incalculable, he fell upon an individuality whom it is much easier to define by opprobrious names than to classify in a calm and scientific spirit. (100)

Interestingly, Robert Siegle has found that in the original serial version of *Chance* (published in the Sunday magazine sections of the *New York Herald* from 21 January to 30 June 1912), the governess "had been early married and soon widowed" (84), but that Conrad omitted these details in the later book printing. The inclusion of her marriage history would have placed the governess more firmly within the strictly monogamous value conventions of middle-class domesticity. Conrad, however, renders ambiguous such an easy assimilation. For, though the governess "(out of a nobleman's family) [was] so judiciously selected (a lady, and connected with well-known country people as she said) to direct the studies, guard the health, form the mind, polish the manners, and generally play the perfect mother to that luckless child" (98), she is tainted, during the family tragedy, with a questionable morality exemplified in an act of theft. What is more, the items that she steals ("a jewelled penholder, an ivory and gold paper knife, . . . some chased silver boxes presented by de Barral" [98]) are particularly representative of the status of the middle class in the heart of the home. The theft highlights how the symbols of middle-class status could be artificially assumed, how the middle-class home was itself indefensible, penetrable from within by a moral failure.

The governess in *Chance* is a partial substitution, a replacement that ironizes, by repeating with a difference, the authorization of middle-class ideal domesticity in the moral institution of motherhood. Because Flora's governess demonstrates her difference from the ideal of (middle-class) moral femininity, she is only a mockery, "the trick of a 'perfect lady' manner (severely conventional) and the soul of a remorseless brigand" (93). The fakeness of the femininity—as a source and model of morality—that suffuses the governess's characterization in *Chance* is constructed through her contingency to the production of a commodity world, within a broad operative field of rising capitalism, speculation, and the growing instabilities of industrial labor markets. In this, the governess in *Chance* references the social history of the professionalization of women's work, which was becoming a focus of concern in the latter part of the nineteenth century. The Victorian governess became a central point of discussion for those who sought for a change in the relation between gender and waged labor, and eventually between gender and the professions, through her plight as a woman in-between, of a woman both inside and outside domestic relations.[8] What happened with the influx of governesses into middle-class homes was a schism in the conceptualization of motherhood, where motherhood and its internal grounding in natural instincts and natural morality were exposed as subject to forces of production and consumption, supply and demand. The paradox of the governess was that in order to educate children of the middle to upper classes, she had to be a middle-class woman herself, for only then would she infuse her charges, by her mere presence, with the morality proper to their social standing. As Mary Poovey explains, "Positioning the governess against a normative definition of woman as wife and mother reinforced [a] complex ideological system. . . . This juxtaposition shored up the distinction between (abnormal) women who performed domestic (in this case maternal) labor for wages and those who did the same work for free, as an expression of a love that was generous, non-competitive, and guaranteed by the natural force of maternal 'instinct'" (144).

The governess in *Chance* shows that middle-class women did not naturally embody middle-class morality; class position could therefore be faked. The novel reveals fakeness in the governess' version of middle-class morality by sexualizing her. The circumstances into which the governess fell, by virtue of her economic dependence on men who had fallen, argues Poovey, were interpreted by Lady Easterlake in her 1844 critique of Jane Eyre as drawing an authoritative and God-given, distinction between the lady of leisure and the governess. What differentiated the governess, Easterlake contended, were the signs of "vulgarity" associated with the working class and, specifically, with the overabundance of sexual knowledge that was identified with working-class women through their exposure to the public sphere.

The Victorian governess is an ambivalent figure because she, by doubling the mother, invokes the repressed class imbalances and contradictions at the heart of middle-class identities. Reminiscent of the governess who tries to possess Flora, the little girl in Henry James's *The Turn of the Screw* (1897), the governess in *Chance,* the wage-earning woman, was characterized with "manly" features and signs of sexual difference that marked her with an aggressive, lascivious sexuality. Such gender crossing and lasciviousness manifested, as Anne McClintock says, degenerate features that depended on colonial narratives.

The governess, Marlow assures in *Chance,* is not a figure of excessive sexuality, though she "harboured a secret taste for patronizing young men of sorts—of a certain sort" and was suspected of being "an artificial, heartless, vulgar-minded woman with the lowest possible ideals" (73). She did not speculate upon marrying de Barral. Yet, her years of practiced and "constant self-repression" (104) did not preclude her from "the fires of the most abandoned passion" (105), "something like an emanation of evil from her eyes" (116), a passion that proves her, Marlow insists, "capable ... of walking backwards into a precipice" (103):

> Do you look upon governesses as creatures above suspicion or necessarily of moral perfection? I suppose their hearts would not stand looking into much better than other people's. Why shouldn't a governess have passions, all the passions, even that of libertinage, and even ungovernable passions; yet suppressed by the very same means which keep the rest of us in order; early training—necessity—circumstances—fear of consequences; till there comes an age, a time when the restraint of years becomes intolerable—and infatuation irresistible? (103)

What arouses the irresistible infatuation, the passion, in the governess is precisely the arrival of her "supposed nephew," Charley. The plan, which the governess instigates, is that Charley will seduce sixteen-year-old Flora and that he will run off with the governess once the inheritance has been won. The play of incest between the governess and her nephew reveals illicit female sexuality and the knowledge of it, underlying and threatening with inauthenticity the moral fiber of motherhood on which middle-class power relies. The moral rectitude of motherhood here becomes a perversity, a refuge of illicit passions, replicated in the vulgar world of incest, love affairs, and thieving. It is in the place of her sexuality and passion—in the place where she is shown as thieving, mimicking, and transforming middle-class respectability—that the governess' world comes to represent the "ungovernable."

The Victorian governess and her plight became a central concern precisely because she was the mother who got paid for performing the duties that should have come naturally to her, revealing that femininity, in its most natural form, was a construction in flux of the market and, in all of its natural morality, essentially corrupt and deceptively staged. In *Chance,* money—a credit system where the referents of investment are evanescent or fraudulent—assumes the same symbolic function of the name of the father, which is changeable, unstable, and often unrecognized. The sailors call him "Mr. Smith," the name the Fynes chose for Flora to camouflage her family origins when de Barral was publicly demoralized. "Was he a foreigner?" the unnamed narrator ruminates. "It's clearly a French name. I suppose it *was* his name?" (70). Marlow answers by referring to de Barral's allegation to Scottish heritage but rejoins, "every great man has done that" (70), putting into question the name itself, its certainty of lineage, and its stake in the processes of legible signification.[9]

Indeed, the governess in *Chance* represents, in the home, the fraud the text exhibits as fundamental to the economies of thrift constituent of the middle-class public sphere and the market in which the father is engaged. The Victorian governess was actually, as Katheryn Hughes has shown, a product of such aberrations, corruptions, and moral failures in middle-class market relations and institutions. Fortunes made quickly could be lost just as quickly due to rising capital investments, speculation, and industrialization; thus, a family rising in the middle classes could fall into destitution, leaving unmarried daughters, like Flora, sorely in need of an alternative source of income. Hughes writes, "Fraudulent 'men of business' . . . served to deprive women who had been left reasonably secure from enjoying their economic independence. . . . In cases like these, where the family was 'reduced from extreme affluence to extreme distress,' there was no choice but to send the girls out as governesses immediately" (28–29). In *Chance,* the governess's thefts within the home are parallel to the public crimes of de Barral, the rising man of business. "He's nothing but a thief," the governess cries (122), "carrying out," adds Marlow, "transactions of an intimate nature and of no moral character" (75). However, de Barral's transgression was to have made a mockery of the word "thrift," and the whole system of money and circulation in which the enterprise was engaged, by emptying it of meaning and flaunting it as an item for sale, taking money for it when there was nothing there to buy. The savings that de Barral's publicity promises are nothing but deception, the illusion of prominent capital backing empty of signification, "mere names" (79), morally bankrupt. The advertising he sold was filled with phony promises and cheap allusions to investment opportunities that did not exist.

De Barral's criminal venture into advertising and speculation exposed that in middle-class commodity culture, names were irrelevant, deceptive, devoid of the references they were supposed to assure. Furthermore, because de Barral had fallen from the class standing that he had "played," he is an intruder, even an impostor, in the middle-class economy, just as the Victorian governess portrayed in *Chance* is also "artificial" (73), a player in the middle-class home, only a simulation of the real, the "God-given," in motherhood, valuing the artificiality of money speculation over the name with its assurances of natural morality. Both de Barral and the governess come to represent the already fallen structure internal to the middle class, evoking the specter of both the market and the underclass, of the "falseness" and "fallenness," the economic precariousness, inside the familial, social, gender, and economic conventions of the Victorian middle class.

By likening de Barral's plight to the fate of the governess, *Chance* exemplifies what Anne McClintock has discerned as a last-ditch defensiveness of a paternal authority weakened in colonial encounters. De Barral's inheritance, the security of his family's financial and social position, are shattered. Interestingly, the falseness and failures of de Barral's business ventures, his advertising, and his pretensions to middle-class identity, result from investments in colonial enterprises which turn out to evaporate, or to be based on absurd financial grounding or false pretenses:

> Under the name of that institution de Barral ... had been financing an Indian prince who was prosecuting a claim for immense sums of money against the government. It was an enormous number of scores of lakhs—a miserable remnant of his ancestors' treasures—that sort of thing. And it was all authentic enough. There was a real prince; and the claim too was sufficiently real—only it was not a valid claim.... He had gone in for the most

> fantastic schemes: a harbour and docks on the coast of Patagonia, quarries in Labrador—such-like speculations. Fisheries to feed a canning factory on the banks of the Amazon was one of them. A principality to be bought in Madagascar was another. (80–81)

In *Chance*, colonial capitalism is the ultimate referent of middle-class economic de-authentication, de-authorization, and the source of its moral collapse from within.

Significantly, Victorian discourse on the moral aberrations of governesses also tended to link the moral falseness of the governess's mothering to colonial situations, as the Jane Eyre example would demonstrate. Ann Laura Stoler has shown how nursemaids and governesses in the Indies were seen as ideal bourgeois bodies subject to racial contamination. "In the Netherlands," she writes, "a new science of domestic medicine warned *burgerlijk* mothers against leaving their children's rearing to such 'lowly beings,' exhorting them to manage their children's bodies in ways that would both protect them *and* ensure that middle-class women would stay at home" (1995: 154). For instance, masturbation was something, a 1898 handbook by a colonial doctor proclaimed, which resulted from the "extremely pernicious" (155) moral influence of native servants. Just as de Barral's project is shown as morally bankrupt in its connections to the colonies, the governess's morality is shown as pure trickery in its allusions to sexuality. The parallels established in the text between de Barral's plight and the governess's—their interlocking "falls" within the middle class—link her sexualization to his colonial investments. Both are represented as empty mockeries of middle-class styles, particularly ideas about gender that framed what it meant to be middle class.

When the governess departs, Flora, too, falls upon the necessity of becoming a governess to earn an income. More important, however, it is Mrs. Fyne who comes to replace the governess, for the two are repeatedly compared: "A something which was not coldness, nor yet indifference, but a sort of peculiar self-possession gave her [Mrs. Fyne] the appearance of a very trustworthy, very capable and excellent governess" (41). And later, "Inside, at the table bearing the lamp, we saw Mrs. Fyne sitting with folded arms and not a hair of her head out of place. She looked exactly like a governess who had put the children to bed; and her manner to me was just the neutral manner of a governess" (50). And again, "There is a certain amount of what I would politely call unscrupulousness in all of us. Think for instance of the excellent Mrs. Fyne, who herself, and in the bosom of her family, resembled a governess of a conventional type" (100). Mrs. Fyne's attitude of self-sufficiency, her indifference, her folded arms, mimic the governess who is, ironically, imitating the middle class mother Mrs. Fyne is supposed to be.

In fact, Mrs. Fyne's feminist doctrine, "naïvely unscrupulous" (62), calls for the same kind of unapproachability and egoism as the governess's conduct exhibited. It is, quite succinctly, the doctrine of the governess. It upheld a "feminine free morality" (65–66), advocated acting with no consideration for anyone (58), "a knock-me-down doctrine—a practical individualistic doctrine" (59), which Marlow summarizes thus: "that no consideration, no delicacy, no tenderness, no scruples should stand in the way of a woman . . . from taking the shortest cut towards securing for herself the easiest possible existence. She had even the right to go out of existence without considering any one's feelings or convenience, since some women's existences were made impossible by the short-sighted baseness of men" (59).

In advocating civil and intellectual equality for women, Mrs. Fyne's feminist doctrine seems to describe the plight of the governess as the exemplary woman working for wages, the middle-class woman of independent means. However, Mrs. Fyne's version of feminist independence is devoid of sexuality, and, in fact, sexuality is precisely what Mrs. Fyne resents in Flora. "It is true," says Marlow, "that Mrs. Fyne did not want women to be women. Her theory was that they should turn themselves into unscrupulous sexless nuisances" (189–90). Yet, Marlow continues, Flora offends Mrs. Fyne by using her sexuality for economic solvency, placing money at the center of both domestic love and feminine unscrupulousness: "[Mrs. Fyne] can't forgive Miss de Barral for being a woman and behaving like a woman. And yet this is not only reasonable and natural, but it is her only chance. A woman against the world has no other resources but in herself" (188). Mrs. Fyne's doctrine leads Flora to her fall, as Flora herself explains to Marlow at the scene, "I don't see why I shouldn't be as reckless as I please" (45). Yet, what Flora calls recklessness is her flight away from domestic proprieties and surveillance as she moves toward the increasingly uprooted, open, explosive, and undefinable space of the colonial mission.

Flora leaves the community of Mrs. Fyne's girlfriends in order to marry Anthony, an act Marlow describes as "this other leap" (209), with Flora "afraid to stumble, ready to fall: (337), "near the edge of a ninety-foot sheer drop" (249). Flora's ambivalent relation to middle-class femininity remains a pivotal concern in the text, especially in view of her continued barrenness. The Fynes and especially Mrs. Fyne worry that Anthony is making a mistake in marrying beneath him, opening the home to moral depravity: "The daughter of a poet and the daughter of a convict are not comparable in the consequences of their conduct if their necessity may wear at times a similar aspect. Amongst these consequences I could perceive undesirable cousins for these dear healthy girls, possible causes of embarrassment in the future" (161–62). In fact, Anthony and Flora's marriage and reproduction would disturb the Fynes' own ideal domesticity: "What was distressing ... if I may say so, [was that] the wind of their flight [would disturb] the solemn placidity of the Fynes' domestic atmosphere" (148).

Despite such protests, Flora and Anthony do get married, and Flora, with her just-released father and her newlywed husband, moves on ship. The ship and its internal space, which Anthony decorates to accommodate a lady, repeats and yet subverts the domestic ideal formative of Victorian middle-class homes such as the Fynes'. For though the ship is isolated and contained by a seemingly impenetrable barrier of "uncorruptible waters" (271), it also becomes a structure permeated with the watch of the crew and the interminable gossip that accompanies it, a private space incessantly configured through public talk. "They had the funny, regretful glances, intonations, nods of men who had seen other, better times," says Marlow. "What difference it could have made to the bo'sun and the carpenter Powell could not very well understand. Yet these two pulled long faces and even gave hostile glances at the poop" (286). Circulating around the domestic space that Flora and Anthony have arranged on shipboard, the constant observations and the talk of the crew put into question the authenticity of the conjugal agreement. What Mrs. Fyne had called an act of "duplicity" (157), the secret that Powell calls a "queerness one wouldn't mind" (299), Franklin claims as a source of anxiety, endless speculation, and resentment. The uncertainty and the worry evinced by the crew give the captain's relations with Flora, says Powell, a sense of irreality, of fakeness: "the nature of fairy-tale with a 'they lived happy ever after' termination," of a "light literature ...

[where] the captain of a ship is a remote, inaccessible creature, something like a prince of a fairy-tale" (288).

The domestic space installed for Flora onboard the ship is ambivalently positioned, as Feito says, "between the discourse of the private home and the discourse of History" (184). Exposing the domestic itself—like Flora's unreproductive relations with Anthony—as an inauthentic creation, a technical construction made by dock workers outfitting ships for colonial passage, first mate Franklin says to Powell, "A gang of people from some tip-top West-End house were fussing here on board with hangings and furniture for a fortnight" (297). Here, the colonial narrative directly serves to expose the domestic as a private space opened for public viewing, a mockery of itself, a "floating stage of that tragi-comedy" (272), revealing the moral essence of the lady's bedroom and domestic arrangements to be an empty form.

Flora's ambivalent relation to the reproduction of whiteness destabilizes the operation of femininity as a symbolic coding of racial difference supporting the colonial order. With dynamite onboard, with a collision immanent, in the middle of the night, Powell catches sight of another ship quickly approaching. Losing partially the assurance, certainty, presence, and self-possession of colonial command, Powell cowers and fails to light the flame that would save the ship from a collision between the dark ship and the British trader, the *Ferndale.* From beneath, Flora climbs on deck just as the ocean turbulence erupts onto the surface. Appearing unexpectedly, she grabs from Powell and lights an enormous flare, which will tell the other ship to divert its headlong acceleration: "The flare blazed up violently between them" (318). "And at the same time vanished out of his mind's eye the vision of another flame enormous and fierce shooting violently from a white churned patch of the sea, lighting up the very clouds and carrying upwards in its volcanic rush flying spars, corpses, the fragments of two destroyed ships" (320). The light from the flare marks a visual difference between the two ships, one coming from the colonial islands and one moving toward them with dynamite ready to explode.

The fakeness that characterizes Flora's claims to middle-class domesticity, her trouble with gender, is further represented in her passage to the other side of the colonial border. Flora is uncomfortable with the domestic abode that Anthony is building for her onboard the ship and that she is seeing for the first time. As Feito observes, Flora's sexual subjectivity, because it is constructed around a colonial transfer, changes the domestic ideal into a problem of colonial administration: "If the home is now at risk of being exposed as a disciplinary community by the likes of Mrs. Fyne, then in order to save Flora (and her inheritance) *Chance* must also expose the merchant ship with all its disciplinary procedures, as itself a domestic community" (184–85). Such ambivalence about the borders of the domestic is underscored in Flora's misrecognition of her own image, her reflective transformation into "something the same, *but not quite*," when she comes to inspect what would become her seafaring quarters: "In a dim inclined mirror, Flora caught sight down to the waist of a pale-faced girl in a white straw hat trimmed with roses, distant, shadowy, as if immersed in water, and was surprised to recognize herself in those surroundings" (265). Flora's image here is divided by the eruption of the waters that had, in Powell's fantasy of collision on the border, sprung up from the depths. As the shipmate watches, Flora's identity is here articulated as divided, "alienate[d] from essence" (Bhabha, 1987: 321), the same but different.

For the sake of protecting her father, but against his will, Flora seeks Anthony's protection, choosing to substitute the open spaces of sea travel for the closure of the domestic bedroom. Inside the ship cabin, the perfect charade of domesticity that the decorations in the captain's cabin produce also induces a "home-like effect" (419), like a home but somehow different. The difference resides in the "moral atmosphere, that tension of falsehood, of desperate acting, which tainted the pure sea-atmosphere into which the magnanimous Anthony had carried off his conquest" (415). The suggestion of incest serves to delegitimate a deceptively inflated paternalistic authority as the defense of morality in this passage toward the colonies. The denaturalization—the insinuation of falsified, fraudulent imitations—of bourgeois morality obstructs the resolution, in matrimonial legitimization and reproduction, of narrative desire. *Chance* locates colonial imitation and de-authentication in the de-authorization and destabilization of the bourgeois bedroom—with its contingency to white femininity, middle-class morality, and its symbolization of female reproduction.

Flora's attachment to her father is textually and symbolically invoked as connected to her self-reflectiveness and narcissistic identifications.[10] The second time Flora glimpses herself in the mirror, she and her father are alone in the country. De Barral is trying to convince Flora to "get away" with him: "She had the strength of mind not to spin around [to look at her father]. On the contrary she went on to a shabby bit of mirror on the wall. In the greenish glass her own face looked far off like the livid face of a drowned corpse at the bottom of the pool" (384). This fantasy of a fall is couched in terms that image Flora as a decaying body of disease in dangerous proximity to a nature that would call her back. Referring to Zola's descriptions of Nana's death in disease, Sander Gilman writes, "Nana begins in death to revert to the blackness of the earth, to assume the horrible grotesque countenance perceived as belonging to the world of the black, the word of the 'primitive,' the world of disease" (1985: 105). Nana's death is remarkably similar to what Flora sees in the mirror: "Withered and sunken, they [Nana's cheeks] had taken on the greyish colour of mud, and on that shapeless pulp, in which the features had ceased to be discernible, they already looked like mould from the grave" (44). This association, Gilman goes on, between nature, disease, and raciality, links the biological degradation of racial degeneracy to the hypersexuality of the prostitute, the demimondaine, the working-class woman.

De Barral's moral incertitude undermines his paternal authority. The father's presence, and yet his powerlessness to command, create the suspense and the ambivalence in the plot, the narrative tension and irresolvability, over Flora's reproductiveness. The moral incertitude and ambiguities within domestic space on the ship are bracketed through de Barral's continued efforts to "get away" with his daughter, to hold onto her, by poisoning Anthony. Penetrating from behind the curtain, the father's impressionistically rendered hand—"[Powell] was startled to observe tips of fingers fumbling with the dark stuff. Then they grasped the edge of the further curtain and hung on there, just fingers and knuckles and nothing else" (417)—which surreptitiously breaks through the edges of the captain's room, dispenses the poison in Anthony's cup of brandy, appearing white but unsteady, ghostly, senile, controlled, and fantastic (417), in the dark. The struggle between de Barral and Anthony in the captain's cabin, the rivalry over Flora's fate, indicates that the problem with Flora's reproduction is also the problem of colonization.

The primal scene of murder is narrated as an anecdotal account of the young Powell's attempts to get an overview—to capture in the look, through a skylight—of what is going on in that bedroom below. However, instead of getting a full and coherent view, his sight is partially obstructed by windows, curtains, walls, chairs, lamps, and similar accouterments, creating an impressionistic effect of what should, ordinarily, be a private domestic life. Powell's fascination with watching the scene unfolding is, Marlow explains, caused by his wonder at the unfamiliarity and unease of a place that should affect "the solitude, the peace . . . the safe aspect of familiar things" (419). Powell's obsession with seeing, confounded in his failure to see, creates an insecure erotic space that refuses clear delineations and legibility. In the famous primal memory of the little boy witnessing his parents' sex acts in Freud's case history of the Wolf Man (1918), "the event of which he was a witness was an act of violence" (202), which aroused castration anxiety in his recognition of his mother's difference. Reminiscent of this scene, Powell's watch over the bedroom, and recognition of Flora's difference in her sexual abstinence, serves to figure the text's movement away from the familiarity of the metropolis and toward the uncanny strangeness of the foreign.

Flora's entrance in this fated night into Anthony's living space, where the crime is committed, occurs at the same time as the narrative unexpectedly notes Anthony's African origin: "She looked a child; a pale-faced child with big blue eyes and a red mouth a little open showing a glimmer of white teeth. . . . I [Powell] had never seen them so near to each other before, and it made a great contrast. It was wonderful, for with his beard cut to a point, his swarthy, sunburnt complexion, thin nose and his lean head there was something African, something Moorish in Captain Anthony" (423–24). The sudden appearance of Anthony as African concurs with Flora's sudden crossing of the bedroom threshold, where Anthony appears as uncontrollably full of beastly passion: "I thought Captain Anthony was a man of iron till I saw him suddenly fling his head to the right and to the left fiercely, like a wild animal at bay not knowing which way to break out" (422). Representing reproductive femininity as produced in the passage toward the colonies, Flora's sexual capitulation to her husband, as her father dies, conveys the birth of Anthony's image as black: "Captain Anthony, swarthy as an African, by the side of Flora whiter than the lilies" (427). The end of paternal control resides in the end of purity in sexually segregated racial identities. Inside Flora's womb, in the private recesses, shadowed in night, of the body of the ship, Anthony's blackness spectrally surfaces.

With the symbolic and legally sanctioned foreclosure of interracial unions, the continuity of the colonial power was, in Conrad's work, destabilized in stories of precarious reproduction and weakened paternal authority. The certainty of the colonizer's reproductive legacy through the domestic control of his women would, at least provisionally, ensure a symbolic economy, the certain dissemination of his authority, heritage, and name. The endless indeterminacy that feminine sexuality actually introduced into the policing structures of colonial authority, however, suspends the implementation of colonial rule through domestic authority. The "ghost" that Terry Castle sees as textually marking the lesbian through disruptions in the feminine (where the lesbian emerges only to disappear) is represented in *Chance*—as in *Almayer's Folly* and *An Outcast of the Islands*—through the impossible regulation of female sexuality, the phantom colonial border that continues to make and unmake the domestic resolution of colonial narrative.

Carpentier's Marvelous Conception

> *It was a pure profile from brow to nose, but suddenly, below these proud, impassive features, the mouth turned full and sensual, with lean cheeks rising toward the ear, the strongly modeled lineaments set in a frame of thick black hair held in place, here and there, by celluloid combs. Several races had met in this woman: Indian in the hair and cheekbones, Mediterranean in brow and nose, Negro in the heavy shoulders and the breadth of hips I noticed as she stood up to put her bundle and umbrella in the luggage rack. There was no question but that the living sum of races had an aristocracy of her own.*
>
> —Alejo Carpentier, *The Lost Steps*

In Cuba, as well as in Latin America generally, the idea of racial mixture, originated in conquest and colonialism, has been the center of political and revolutionary speculations since the early nineteenth century. A century ago, José Martí envisioned a philosophy of nation through an image of sexual union across races, emblematized in "nuestra América mestiza": "With the rosary as our guide, our heads white and our bodies mottled, boy Indian and Creole, we fearlessly entered the world of nations" (88). Following Martí, the eminent social and cultural critic Roberto Fernández Retamar transformed the image into other scenes of national integration and vitalism. Retamar claims the "law of evolution"—the mixing of forms—as the source and inspiration of a vast field of creative cultural production and the basis of cultural autonomy.

The philosophies of *mestizaje* allow that the symbolism of adaptation serves to frame the stories of nations founded in the colonial clash of races and global power shifts. The rise of the nation assumes an assimilation into global modernity. In turn, this assimilation implies a national culture that is autonomous, vibrant, and competitive, thus redeemed from labels of anti-progress and technological backwardness. At the center of these tales of national origin sits Madre America, both virgin and victim, the redemptive figure of the multiracial society being born, like a species, as a new culture and the potential of a new type of liberatory cultural expression. Although such reconfigurations of evolution rely on metaphors of reproduction for their narratives of cultural transformation, they also are constantly deferring reproductive closure and fertility. As a result, the progress of the nation is often staged as a desire for the feminine, a desire for seduction that would circulate as the foundational moment. "We set out to conquer freedom," declares Martí, "under the banner of the Virgin" (88). In Martí's vision, the village of America is formed through an initial rivalry where "the conceited villager . . . humiliate[s] the rival who stole his sweetheart" (84). The virgin continent motivates the cultural and intellectual progress that would become the strength and foundation of our America *mestiza*, the triumphant and beautiful nation. At the same time, America is sculpted, in Martí's famous essay, as a crisis, an illness, in motherhood—"Only those born prematurely are lacking in courage" (85)—with the cure being a return to a Latin American masculinity, a competitive masculinity professed through a visionary defiance.

Mestizaje continued to be a central thematic in defining Latin American nationhood through literary production and its aesthetics of innovation. Importing modernist ideas into Cuban letters, Alejo Carpentier, for example, developed his theory of the "lo real maravilloso americano" as a result of evolutionary reproduction: "mix of styles in one and the same work, mix which corresponds to the diverse origins of each style" (González Echevarría, 1985: 37), "mix of elements from diverse cultural traditions, which reveal themselves as artificial when entering into contact with each other and which, together, are a type of summary baroque of the artificial" (38).[1] Between the banality and the repetitions of an atrophied Western artistic tradition and the inspired rejuvenation in the cultural landscapes of the Americas, where Carpentier "discovered" "lo real maravilloso," "there had to be a rupture" (37), a new birth, an emergent and autonomous species. In *The Lost Steps* (1956) (*Los pasos perdidos* [1953]), Carpentier envisions this rupture, the difference between the European avant-garde and what would become Latin American magic realist aesthetics, in terms of Latin America's privileged histories of chance encounters and cultural mixing, the emerging of "the new" in the racial identities formed initially through colonial contacts. Idealized and eroticized, the central character described above—Rosario—is the lure to an original new culture, the first of its kind, and stronger than the degenerate arts of a Europe in demise. The literature of the new nation would be a mixture of local images, indigenous traditions, and universal artistic forms. It would merge through reproduction and give birth to something truer, more passionate and sensual, symbolizing the ascendant competitiveness of the new nation in imagining itself as a culture of difference.

Carpentier's "lo real" serves to mark the severance of Latin American from European artistic traditions. Carpentier would create "the real" of Latin American essential difference as emerging through hybrid forms. Femininity in *The Lost Steps* operates as a site where Carpentier could replicate modernist traditions and also where a regionalized primitive aesthetic could define racial difference as Latin American artistic novelty. Thus sexuality, especially sexuality in women, marks a pivotal concern within Carpentier's racialized discourse of artistic and autochthonously American experimentation. In *The Lost Steps,* the borders between national and racial differences are constructed through feminine identities—virginal, extramarital, homosexual, and interracial—that delay reproduction. In this chapter, I consider how Carpentier's "lo real maravilloso americano"—as the seed, a provisional origin, an instigator of what would develop into a kind of postcolonial theory—evoked feminine sexuality both to create and to bridge the temporal/spatial distance between the modernist subject and the essentially separate foundation of a "new" American artistic tradition.

As a precursor to the idea of the postcolonial, Martí, too, set in motion an emancipatory agenda for the utterance of difference, particularly in terms of imagining a new and more just set of institutional practices. Martí was writing when Cuba was breaking away from Spain, abolishing slavery, and setting up a newly independent social and political entity with its own philosophies, traditions, autochthonous organizations, and character—in short, a new nation. For Marti, then, the very idea of the nation would be transformative. So, what could possibly be the problem in employing metaphors of an aggressively competitive masculinity as an incentive to revolutionary action and national formation? The idea that the nation and the nationalist rhetoric supporting it is shaped through masculinist assumptions will lead to the new nation being formed as an exclusion of the feminine. There are a number of possible repercussions in treating the national as resolutely masculine. For instance, when more than 70 percent of the world's poverty is constituted by women, the interests of the poor get relegated to the periphery of national concern, even while "national interests" or "national security" surface as displays of militaristic and territorial prowess. As Anne McClintock argues, "If nationalism is not transformed by an analysis of gender power, the nation-state will remain a repository of male hopes, male aspirations and male privilege" (385). Women's interests, such as health care, schooling, child care, land reform, world poverty, are characteristically struck from the map defining "the national" or, at the very least, are relegated to subordinated positions within nationalist plans for social change.

In both feminist and nationalist oppositional discourses, the figure of the cross-breeding, culturally migrant woman recalls evolutionary stories in which female sterility allows for transformative possibilities. Recent feminist cultural criticism on Latin America, for example, has tried to recuperate the mixed-blood woman as a lexicon through which contesting narratives of the modern nation are written. Norma Alarcón, for example, commenting on recent Mexican and Chicano literatures, has said that Malintzin, the indigenous woman who translated for Cortés and who, within the stories of Mexican nationalism, gave birth to the first mestizos, portrays "the belief that literature is the intention, through the power of language, to recover memory by recovering the word and to project a future by possessing the word" (283). As a figure of conquest and as a legendary victim of the rape through which the Mexican nation was founded, La Malinche/Malintzin is, for Alarcón, a "producer of history" (286), of agency and opposition, the condition of narratives and of literature, "a redeeming figure, one who will not be still until she is recognized as patriarchy's suppressed woman, the one upon whose body Western civilization has been built" (289). Such criticism supposes that the overfamiliar binaries of Western metaphysics—man/woman, West/rest, subject/object, signifier/signified—are deconstructed *tout court* in the figure of the cross-breeding woman who then can reclaim, automatically, the possibility of resistance to linguistic and therefore political objectifications.

What allows cross-breeding to be read as a progressive opening into the modern in such discourses of oppositionality and emancipation? How does such a symbol get formulated as inspiring a romance of freedom, and whose interests get served by it? Reading *The Lost Steps,* Vera Kutzinski applies Eve Sedgwick's theory of the homosocial to argue that "*mestizaje* becomes legitimated as an exclusively male project or achievement in which interracial, heterosexual rape can be refigured as a fraternal embrace across color ... lines and, significantly, across a female body absented by rape" (168). Femininity is here troped exclusively as the violent meeting-ground between races of men. Kutzinski continues, "The mulatta may be *the* signifier of Cuba's unity-in-racial-diversity, but she has no part in [it]. For the mestizo nation is a male homosocial construct premised precisely upon the disappearance of the feminine" (165). Femininity brings the memory and the history of colonialism into literature, reconstructing a very political and violent meeting of races as an aesthetic product. Femininity contingently ensures ideologically the sustainability of contracts between men, contracts that affiliate nations in the interests of trade and provide the groundwork for global competition. Yet, recognizing that there is, indeed, a political economy of gender, *mestizaje* can be used as a hard-core justification for social injustices, an ideological shield endorsing economic imbalances and practices of domination, even annihilating certain sectors of the population in the interests of a fuller integration into an expanding capitalist system.

Historically, cross-breeding has been a site of political, even oppressive, intervention both by the church and the state as Latin American nations have tried to identify and regulate their populations, instituting economic and social hierarchies while granting and ensuring power to small groups of elites. Sex between races has therefore been a site where new powers of capital defined social relations and where new alliances were formed to set the framework for trade across borders. Originally in Latin America, "purity of blood" was a religious category, signifying untainted Christian belief (Stolcke, 1989). The Spanish nobility in the peninsula opposed the Inquisition's opposition to the "purity of blood" doctrine, as the nobility had mixed with the Jews and the Moors before the Reconquest. In the Americas, the Spanish crown at first tried to institute policies of separation, setting up a "República de españoles" and a "Repúplica de indios," and prohibiting communication and marriage between the two (Mörner, 43). Because of the crown's inability to enforce separateness, and also because of the growing population of mestizos, such policies did not work; as early as 1501, the Spanish monarchy was permitting intermarriage. In fact, intermarriage between the Spanish and Indian nobilities was encouraged, beginning in 1503, as a technique of assimilation (Mörner, 26). "Purity of blood" would be extended to the nobles of the indigenous peoples who converted. It also became, in the eighteenth and nineteenth centuries, a category that the church used to prohibit marriage between unequals (Stolcke, 1989). As Michael Taussig summarizes, "From the sixteenth century onward, sexual intercourse as well as cohabitation between colonizing men and native women in Latin America was not uncommon and was the obvious source of the (in many places numerically dominant) mestizo fraction of the population. Balboa had his beautiful Indian mistress on the Isthmus, and it was poor Spanish men who, living with Indian women, established the European presence across the length and breadth of the Spanish New World.... Here the outstanding feature is the male-controlled access to the women ... and the consequent investment of these women with an extraordinary colonial aura" (182).

Presently, "mixed race" is used as a rhetorical buzzword that slides the very idea of a postcolonial nationhood straightaway into the conceptual framework of global capitalist competition. In other words, the idea of mobility, which is central to the political circulation of cross-breeding—say, the belief that identities are constructable and therefore changeable—also becomes a justification for a furtherance of an aggressive capitalist agenda, projecting a message that the economy is open and accessible, manageable and transforming, offering equitable opportunities for everybody and the possibility of moving around into ever more vital economic positions, a guarantee of free and universal competition between nations. In addition, the breaking down of the borders of identity—a process that a redemptive, even deconstructive, oppositional politics has attributed as a positive feature to hybridity—can translate into the crossing of national borders that a global capitalist expansion performs, and even into a rightist defense for a severe neoliberalization of developing national economies, a breaking down of borders evinced by a complete deregulation of national market protections in the interests of multinational integration. One wonders, indeed, on what terms and in what circumstances the idea of changeability—so central to a poststructural undermining of the modernist master narratives of humanism and human emancipation—becomes embedded within a capitalist ideology of competition and transformation as indicative of increasing market saturation. Indeed, global capitalism has thoroughly reorganized the idea of the transient identity in, for example, the ephemerality of noncontracted labor and decreasing job security—a cultural condition that Stanley Aronowitz and others have called "post-work"—especially in this age of expansive immigration caused by economic and political desperation, the technologization of the work force and the growth of service industries. For Aronowitz, "The bottom is falling out and with it our sense of well-being. . . . For many, recent economic and political developments point to the withering away of comfortable full-time jobs 'with a future.'' . . . What does the term 'globalization' mean for the average working person? . . . Much work keeps flowing out of the country, replaced by temporary, part-time and contingent work, which statisticians optimistically call 'jobs'" (31–34). The exportation of industry and manufacturing out of the United States has affected the conditions of work in other sites, particularly those south of the border, where it is evident that after NAFTA, working conditions and longevity have deteriorated along with the spending power of the working classes, the well-being of citizens, the legitimacy of currencies, and the financial stability of governments. One wonders, too, therefore, whether it is possible (or worth it) now to "resignify" the very notion of mobility and adaptability—"resignify," in Judith Butler's sense of the word, for a feminist reappropriation not merely linguistic but instead leading to a stronger oppositional politics.

With its possible links to the politics of capital flow, it can actually be dangerous to consider hybridity as liberating just because it seems to rip apart a linguistic determinacy or deracinate a positivistic stabilizing of identities—racial, ethnic, economic, or other. Like Carpentier, Néstor García Canclini has analyzed the importing of technologies and other products of modernity into Latin American countries as a potentially creative and emancipatory situation. What he notices is the breaking down of cultural borders, giving rise to an exciting mixture of traditions—indigenous and foreign, ancestral and innovative, artisanal (peasant, popular, craft) and high art—coming into contact with one another in new urban neighborhoods mostly composed of migrants. For Canclini, the antifoundationalism of postmodern philosophies, as well as the iterability of postmodern identities, makes possible cultural syntheses without hierarchies. Like the unnamed narrator of *The Lost Steps,* Canclini celebrates the transnationalization of traditional cultures and their adoption into mass media, arguing that market forces can and do increase international recognition and the commercial potentials of the popular, thereby increasing their profitability and the survival rates of the poor, the rural, and the indigenous. Peasant markets here guarantee freedom. What is missing in Canclini's account is a sense that multinational appropriations are not equitable or just. When AeroPeru, for example, adopted an Amazonian death mask as its company insignia, the indigenous peoples whose symbol it was did not celebrate their recognition as part of a multinational commercial scheme but instead avoided association with airplanes heralding death. In Canclini's view, there is an almost utopic space of cultural integration, a field where players enter freely and compete evenly, responding to commercial desire on the level of the international even while negotiating power. Says Jameson, "García Canclini's work thus gives ammunition to the most vital utopian visions of our own time, of an immense global urban intercultural festival without a center or even any longer a dominant cultural mode. I myself think this view needs a little economic specificity and is rather inconsistent with the quality and impoverishment of what has to be called corporate culture on a global scale" (1998: 66).

Canclini's global carnival of crossing cultures does not account for global corporatism as an insidious force with annihilistic propensities, as well as his elevation of modernization as a compelling and assured road to universal cultural improvement, a tendency to which Carpentier also falls prey. In Canclini's vision, everybody has the chance to move up, and modernization fundamentally benefits everybody:

> Not only did this modernization expansion not succeed in erasing folklore, but many studies reveal that in the last few decades traditional cultures *have*

> *developed by being transformed.* This growth is the result of at least four types of causes: (a) the impossibility of incorporating the entire population into urban industrial production; (b) the need of the market to include traditional symbolic structures and goods in the mass circuits of communication in order to reach even the popular layers least integrated into modernity; (c) the interest of political systems in taking folklore into account with the goal of strengthening their hegemony and legitimacy; (d) continuity in the cultural production of the popular sectors. (153)

However, as Chandra Mohanty has pointed out, the labor of craft production in the global economy does not equitably give access to those heretofore neglected segments of traditional and popular cultures, and does not redeem, through legitimization, the economically marginal. In fact, Mohanty has shown, through her analysis of Mexican women's labor, how craft production has been complicit in relegating women in particular to less lucrative and more exploitable positions in the processes of production. Working in "leisure time" in their homes, female workers in the craft industry have been easily underpaid and denied contracts and benefits because of the way they can fall under the label of domestic economies and therefore outside of the main, integral sites of industrial manufacturing: "Ideologies of domesticity, femininity, and race form the basis of the construction of the notion of 'women's work' for Third-World women in the contemporary economy. . . . Ideas of *flexibility, temporality, invisibility,* and *domesticity* in the naturalization of categories of work are crucial in the construction of Third-World women as an appropriate and cheap labor force" (20). The definition of Third World women's work as domestic has eased a capitalist strategy for recolonizing the poor. Clearly, hybrid cultures have not been sites of liberation for everybody.

It is not just media representation and recognition that is at stake here. For example, a recent hurricane in Central America sent many into flight. The death toll was high, and the widespread destruction to property also destroyed the means of livelihood for some of the poorest populations in the world. The event was covered prolifically by the mass news media, spurring efforts of humanitarian aid by both the private and public sectors, not-for-profits, nongovernmental organizations, national and international relief efforts, international and federal public assistance programs. Concurrently, the president of the United States paid a visit to the Central

American region to express his solidarity with the hurricane victims and the governments and the humanitarian relief efforts that have been trying to ease the pain and economic desperation resulting from the widespread damage. His message was one of hope and support. But at the same time, the U.S. president propounded his agenda of renegotiating the debts of Central American nations and implementing government austerity measures in conformity with the guidelines of the International Monetary Fund and the World Bank. This agenda would open Central America to wider penetration by U.S. production, liberalize the economy for U.S. manufacturing interests, and broaden the market for U.S. consumer goods, thus setting the course for the spread of NAFTA. Migrancy here has become an excuse for capitalist domination.

The widespread media recognition of marginal and migrant populations in this event has not, therefore, led to an increasing economic viability of their popular expressions but rather has paved the road to further misery. People do not become migrants to make TV shows more interesting or colorful, nor does everyone end up more happy and beautiful when Avon sells its make-up to indigenous peoples in the Amazon, nor do rural cultures benefit when Benetton puts their photographs on T-shirts. Having "voice" and representation in media and academic discourse does not solve the problem of economic desperation or the squeezing out by capital of ever more distant corners of the world population.

What Canclini's view bypasses is the kind of complex critiques of cultural corporatism and hybridization that, for example, Clarice Lispector, in her novel *The Hour of the Star,* has been able to work through in relation to the popular in Brazil. As a migrant from the impoverished Northeast, Lispector's protagonist Macabéa is not only completely out of tune with the ways the media in the novel speak about popular culture but is also in the process of being run down by the commercial internationalization of the popular. She is, in short, unrepresented and unrepresentable. Ugly, diseased Macabéa is dying on a diet of Coca-Cola and hot dogs while dreaming of becoming Marilyn Monroe; addicted to advertisements, she is craving a meal of cold cream when she gets run over by a Mercedes-Benz in a hit-and-run accident and bleeds to death on the sidewalk. "The record that is about to begin," explains Lispector, "is written under the sponsorship of the most popular soft drink in the world even though it does not earn me anything; a soft drink that is distributed throughout the world. It is the same soft drink that sponsored the recent earthquake in Guatemala. Despite the fact that it tastes of nail polish, toilet soap and chewed plastic. None of this prevents people from loving it with servility and subservience" (23). It is clear that Macabéa's life is neither included in symbolic structures nor in mass circuits of communication, nor is it necessary for the perpetuation of national hegemonies but instead is neglected and overrun by them, quite literally crushed.

Unlike Canclini, Lispector is able to show the complete abjection and alienation of the poor caused by globalization and how this abjection creates, as Cixous says, "death in the quotidian, the insignificant, the ordinary" (141). Macabéa's problem is not only that she is a typist but that she is a bad typist and hence basically a waste or a wounding of the profit nexus that Canclini celebrates as the cause of cultural migration, national integration, and mixing. Macabéa is shown as the unrecognizable within capitalism because she is virtually unhirable; as female labor, she has no value to exchange. She is, as well, an orphan and a virgin, and her nonexchangeability on the sexual level is intertwined with her economic obsolescence. "But the person whom I am about to describe," comments Lispector, "scarcely has a body to sell; nobody desires her, she is a harmless virgin whom nobody needs" (14). Here, the eroticization of globalism through the intensified sexiness of the commodity—as Jameson says, "the reason so many people now feel that this boring and archaic thing is sexy" (69)—comes to an end in Macabéa, exposing an aporia, a gap between capital flows, the seduction of consumerisms and systems of exchange on the one hand and, on the other, the struggle to exist. Lispector portrays how, in short, a corporate taking-over of culture has made the human unusable and devalued—specifically in those populations, like women and the urban poor, which are marginal to the growing service economy focusing on production for international consumption and neoliberal trade. Who ends up crushed under the speeding wheels of the unstoppably mobile, ubiquitous corporate trademark, the commercialization of the popular? Made utterly abject by capitalism, Macabéa is unable to survive in a hybrid world. She is the thorn in the side of Canclini's vision—and also Carpentier's—of global capitalist redemption in the sale and media appropriation of popular cultures where modernity and tradition meet.

"Lo real maravilloso americano," as explored in *The Lost Steps*, is as much a search for the origin, the "essence" of Latin American cultural character in its own singular climate, as a theoretical journey constructing that origin at its endpoint. As such, it moves in a recapitulatory regression of the present through a series of sexual-racial relations, each with its own cultural setting, toward an end that is its own beginning. Race, as a biological discourse embedded in sexual regulations, furnishes the narrative of the stages of artistic development marking parallel time back through the human history of civilization and personal experience. Based loosely on Carpentier's own voyages in search of the source of the Orinoco River in Venezuela, *The Lost Steps* tells of an unnamed narrator's growing alienation in the mechanized and automated world of a decadent, stagnant, and unnamed cosmopolitan city resembling New York. Wandering distractedly through the streets in the dead-time of vacation, the narrator, a director of public relations films, meets by chance the curator of an ethnomusicological museum, an old friend and mentor who gets the university to sponsor him on a trip to the jungle on the commission of finding the most primitive instruments, the origin of music.

The narrator-protagonist sets out with his lover Mouche, an astrologist well influenced by the atrophied intellectual fashions of the day (his wife, Ruth, has already left on tour with her acting company), and arrives in an unnamed Latin American city (a cross between Caracas and Havana) the day before a coup d'état.[2] To escape the confinement of a regulated curfew, the narrator-protagonist and Mouche accept the invitation of a Canadian painter, also staying at the hotel, to her home in Los Altos for the duration of the rebellion. Vexed by his suspicions of the seductions going on between Mouche and the painter, the narrator-protagonist decides to start his trip into the heart of the jungle, meeting along the road Rosario, a *mestiza* native, beautiful in her primitive knowledge of nature, with whom he falls in love. One day, while the women are bathing at the river bank, Mouche breaches the law of the jungle by caressing Rosario's body. Rosario intuitively responds by beating her. Ridding himself of Mouche by sending her back when she contracts malaria directly following her offense, the narrator-protagonist finds the sought-for instruments and resolves to stay permanently in the jungle. However, when the narrator-protagonist, inspired by his proximity to origins (Spanish, the language he speaks with Rosario, is also his mother's language), decides to compose a choral work of the *Odyssey*, he realizes that his project in the jungle depends on a supply of paper and ink. Therefore, when a plane mysteriously appears overhead (Ruth has put out a reward to find him), the narrator-protagonist flags it down and boards it, leaving his score with Rosario as he promises to return after divorcing Ruth and buying notebooks.[3] He does return, only to find that the entrance has been hidden in the rising waters of the rainy season, and that Rosario has been "married" to someone else and is expecting a child.

In *The Lost Steps*, Carpentier reworks the narratives of race that he explored in his earlier novels where racialism, purified through marginality and ritual, provided the energy necessary for a revolutionary literature. In Carpentier's previous writings, primitivism, racial character, and exotic rituals provided a repertoire of symbols for developing regional expression, a way of imagining Latin American artistic production not as just an imitation or repetition of European tradition, where *novelas de la tierra, costumbrista,* and *indígenista* writings were still so embedded. Afro-Antillian Cuban culture was mystified, demarcated, made tendentious, and reified through, for example, long and detailed descriptions of religious music and dance where revolutionary consciousness emerged as opposition to imperializing economies. In his 1927 novel *Ecue-Yamba-O* (which Carpentier himself would later renounce), the vitality of Cuban black ritual and music serves as a bedrock on which the *vanguardista* built an identity of nation. The revolutionary energy emerges through landscape, an American nature surging into a religious and cultural expression of resistance.[4] During, for example, a ñáñigo initiation ceremony, amid stanzas of song and rhythms of chant, dancing bodies possessed by the spirits form circles that rotate around each other, unified through movement and vernacular instrumentation. The fervor and excitement that ensue, "terribly primitive" (195), escalating into frenzy, unroll through blood metaphors linked to the provincial and exuberantly natural setting that opens the novel and that is also invoked in the brewing storm, "clouds of a storm which were closing in over the invisible war" (186), breaking on the outside. Culture, and particularly black underground ritual culture, is irrevocably collapsed into a determining nature, a localized landscaping that sets it in opposition to European aesthetic production.

The romanticism in this early text, formulated within a European positivist tradition,[5] was later displaced by Carpentier's adaptation of a modernist primitivist aestheticism in "lo real maravilloso americano." The omniscience of the narrative in *Ecue-Yamba-O* tended to unify and ontologize racial exoticism as primal revolutionary material open to the operations and speculations of a scientifically observant, rationalizing eye. However, as set out in the introduction to his next novel, *El reino de este mundo* (Kingdom of This World) (1949), Carpentier's new artistic agenda would no longer regard black ritual as a centerpiece, a separate entity, which an objectivist *vanguardista* prose would construct as the material of ethnological description feeding a revolutionary class consciousness. Particularly American racial factors were represented and synthesized by a constant shifting of interpretative perspectives and a weaving of different temporal sites of signification, all coming into the marvelous contradictions of chance encounter. Race was not any longer a circumscribed and singular expression of revolutionary culture but instead a diversity of cultural processes mixing promiscuously. The role of the new American artist was to name forms that would result from the coming together of seemingly antagonistic entities in the cultural landscapes of the Americas:

> When André Masson wanted to draw the jungle of the Martinique island, with the incredible interlacing of its plants and the obscene promiscuity of certain fruits, the marvelous truth of the subject devoured the painter, leaving him a little less than impotent in front of the paper in white (the target). And it had to be a painter from America, the Cuban Wilfredo Lam, who showed us the magic of the tropical vegetation, the unbridled creation of forms from our nature—with all its metamorphoses and symbioses—in monumental canvases of a singular expression in contemporary painting. (As cited in the reissuing of the essay in *Tientos y diferencias* [1967]; see "De lo real maravilloso americano," in *Ensayos*, 113)

The "shock" of surrealism is changed into "lo real" of America through an evolutionary language, a narrative of biodiversity, which gets elided, in turn, into a cultural story of sex: the history of colonialism, and the origin and specificity of a "new," "American" creative act. An initial break into the blank pages of history through potency, passion, and promiscuity, American art is here represented through metaphors of colonial rape woven through the language of evolutionary selection and ascendance.

The artistically "American" act would restore masculine potency, lost to European modernisms, by deploying feminine sexuality as a canvas on which the artist can speak "the new" as evolutionary change, ecological exuberance, racial polyphony, and heterogeneity. Both Oscar Montero and Sylvia Molloy have argued that sexuality and particularly male sexuality played a large role in defining a new tradition of Latin American arts distinguished from a European avant-garde steeped in philosophies of decadence. For Montero, the softness and sensitivity characteristic of Latin American *modernismo* was left out in academic treatments of the movement in favor of an institutionalization of Latin American letters, where the works would be interpreted, in contrast to the moral and linguistic deviations defining European modernisms, as expressions of "intellectual rigor" and "a vaguely neoplatonic sublime" (222). Sylvia Molloy has likewise demonstrated how the importation of modernist ideas into Latin America worked to police gender, remaking cultural strength as a battle against feminization, ill health, softness, and nervous weakness. As in the evolutionary model, situating national identities, in such metaphors of resistance and difference, becomes a matter of developing masculine virtuosity in reproductive competitions, or proving potency against the degeneration of desire signifying literary practice in dominant modernist trends elsewhere. Moving beyond early twentieth-century *modernismo*, Carpentier's fiction still is concerned with affirming national difference in the remasculinization of masculinities shored up in the promise of reproduction. Using evolutionary symbolisms of cross-breeding and constantly deferring domestication, Carpentier represents this process in a constant repositioning of femininity as a barrier that a national subject must access to reproduce itself as difference.

The "new" way of creating art is, Carpentier maintains, a culture of eroticism. As an aestheticized revisioning of first contact and its scenes of rape, the eroticism of "lo real maravilloso americano" is an eroticism that creates monstrous forms, the unusual, through a constant merging of forms and figures. Far from "discovering" the strange in ethnic difference and the ethnographic object, the distinction of "*nuestra historia*," claimed

Carpentier in a 1975 lecture delivered at the Universidad Central de Venezuela, would exhibit that

> this American soil was the theater of the most sensational ethnic encounter which the annals of our planet registered, encounter of the Indian, of the black, and of the European of a size more or less clear, destined, in the future, to mingle, to intermingle symbiosis of cultures, of beliefs, of popular arts, in the most tremendous *mestizaje* which one could ever contemplate. ("Conciencia e identidad de América," 133)

The modernist imperative of the "new" would transpire, in America and its arts, in the creation of monstrous, marvelous forms through a radical and inspirational racial mixture naturally selected. "The ugly, the deformed, the terrible, also can be marvelous. Everything unusual is marvelous" ("Lo barroco y lo real maravilloso" [1975] (1990), 184). Biological signifiers here become indistinguishable from cultural ones. For Latin American culture, the metaphors of symbiosis and fecundity, evoking evolutionary science, are literalized and materialized through Carpentier's insistence on the reality of the biological contradiction against the falsity of European simulation, abstraction, and posturing. As he says in *The Lost Steps*, "And all this, there below, intertwined, tangled, in a grappling, a coupling, monstrous and orgiastic, incests that represent the supreme confusion of forms" (205). And further, "I was asking myself whether perhaps the role of these lands in the history of man might not be to make possible for the first time certain symbioses of cultures" (119–20). The difference of Latin American arts would be situated in "lo real" emphatically registered, through both an espousal and a renunciation of surrealism, in the political history of evolutionary biology overcoming the selective limitations posed by racial mixture.

One way in which Carpentier negotiates the contradiction that his work evinces toward European artistic tradition is by discussing how the privilege of "lo real" distinguishes Latin America from the United States. The difference, which is a difference of the history in colonial practice, is a difference of love. As the example of a nation founded in the name of independence and emancipation, the United States, according to Carpentier, did not succeed in transforming colonial relations of power; the color line, even after slavery, remained as the fundamental obstacle to the freedom of the "new" in racial mixing: "The landlords continue to be the same landlords: the big property-holders, the big merchants continue to live exactly the same as before. It didn't enter in anybody's head that there could have been an emancipation of slaves" ([1979] (1990), 322). The U.S. color line created, in Carpentier's view, an originary prohibition restricting the birth of vital cultures and economies of change, instituting policies of separation that kept identities from transforming. In contrast, in Latin America, the wars of independence resulted in a constant cultural shuffling—a "convivencia" (cohabitation)—between the colonizers and the indigenous racial fabric of the Americas, from which the native "criollo" and, subsequently, the *mestizo* was born. Outside of the sexual taboos instigated by the economies of the U.S. color line, the "mezclarse, entremezclarse" (mixing, intermixing) of free-flowing Latin American passions and cultural commerce created, according to Carpentier, the possibility of freedom and originality—of autonomy, independence, and emancipation from the sterile European histories of nontransmutation, nontransformation, and biological (cultural) repetitions.

Restrictions over access to women furnish Carpentier with multiple possibilities for telling stories of difference—of racial and national difference—as encoded within femininity. In fact, what motivates the plot in *The Lost Steps* is Rosario's continuing infertility and her refusal to marry. Through Rosario's sexual inaccessibility, as she continually stands in the way of closing the novel in a reproductive resolution, the novel stages its tensions and plots, its crises and turns, its journey to the origin. To consecrate the new church, for example, which would be the founding gesture of El Adelantado's most primitive cry at the center of the jungle, Father Pedro insists that the narrator-protagonist marry Rosario. Prohibited from taking vows with Rosario by his marriage to Ruth, the narrator-protagonist contemplates the situation:

> As I prized above everything in the world the loyalty Rosario put into anything connected with me, the thought of deceiving her revolted me, especially in a matter to which a woman instinctively attaches so much importance, who must be assured of a home to shelter the living home of an always possible pregnancy. (223)

Rosario becomes the end toward which the plot, and the narrator-protagonist, must always be gravitating. The narrator-protagonist's quest for the source is directed through, he says, an unrequited desire to impregnate the primitive mother as the origin of language, of art, music and The

Word. "The Mother, with swollen belly, which was at one and the same time breasts, womb, and sex," he ruminates, "the first figure modeled by man, when under his hands the possibility of the object came into being" (183).

Critics have debated whether Rosario represents the continuance of a surrealist tradition or a radical breaking from it. Femininity, for Carpentier's critics, has a double orientation: it allows him to repeat surrealist tradition while also separating from and transforming it. On the one hand, the same can be said of *The Lost Steps* that Torres-Rosaldo observes in the symbolic configuration of Otherness in *El reino de este mundo*: "an analysis which centers on the representation of the woman in the novel shows that she is used by Carpentier as an aesthetic-literary referent with the one intention to recreate the unusual as a basic element for his theory of marvelous reality" (208). Breton's mapping of Paris through the wanderings of the hysterical Nadja can find parallels, for instance, in the narrator-protagonist's mapping, through his desire for Rosario, a recapitulatory cultural history in the jungle. On the other hand, while Nadja's insane wanderings define a new surrealist map with the city at its center, Rosario leads the narrative away from the theaters of the metropolis and toward geographical margins of history narrated in the jungle.

Representations of women and their sexualization—at the heart of surrealism's cult of the unusual—also make, according to the critics, Carpentier's "lo real maravilloso" into an avant-garde movement in opposition to surrealism—a gateway into an oppositional, nationalist aesthetic in the modernist tradition but outside of it.[6] Amaryll Chanady, for instance, points out: "It is simplistic to criticize the Cuban author for imitating metropolitan conventions and identifying with European preoccupations. His concept of the marvelous real acquired an entirely different function from that of the Surrealist marvelous" (137). Chanady goes on to place the representation of women at the center of Carpentier's realignment of surrealist literary practice within a regional aesthetic:

> [Carpentier] coins the expression *lo real maravilloso* in an obvious reference to the French Surrealists' exhortation that reality should be considered as marvelous. And Carpentier's depiction of the female indigenous protagonist in *The Lost Steps* (1953) as a spontaneous, natural woman living in a

community untouched by the corruption of modern society involves a nostalgic utopian recreation of an idealized past indubitably influenced by the European pastoral mode. (137)

In the erotics that specifies "lo real maravilloso americano" in *The Lost Steps,* Rosario occupies the position that catalyzes change, where the narrator-protagonist can see his subjectivity as different. Rosario, paradoxically, obstructs "the unusual" by conceiving it.

In *The Lost Steps,* Carpentier's "lo real maravilloso americano" is beginning to be reimagined, developing into his later aestheticization of America in the baroque. These two artistic movements—"lo real maravilloso" and "lo barroco"—are, indeed, difficult to segregate and compartmentalize. In actuality, they seem to overlap. In "Lo barroco y lo real maravilloso," for example, Carpentier asserts that "The baroque ... manifests itself where there is transformation, mutation, innovation.... America, continent of symbiosis, of mutations, vibrations, of mixings, was always baroque" (179; my translation). In *Explosion in a Cathedral* (1963) (*El siglo de las luces* [1962]), Carpentier repeats the gesture of naming the forms created in interracial crossings:

> Esteban marveled to realize how the language of these islands had made use of agglutination, verbal amalgams and metaphors to convey the formal ambiguity of things which participated in several essences at once. Just as certain trees were called "acadia-bracelets", "pineapple-porcelain", "wood-rib", "ten o'clock broom", "cousin clover", "pitcher-pine-kernal", "tisane-cloud", and "iguana-stick", many marine creatures had received names which established verbal equivocations in order to describe them accurately. Thus a fantastic bestiary had arisen of dog-fish, oxen-fish, tiger-fish, snorers, blowers, flying fish. (178)

Perhaps one of the main characteristics that distinguishes Carpentier's baroque is the complete undoing of the concept of the origin in all of its many guises, a radical and constant shifting of identity and form. As Djelal Kadir contests, "Far from the achievement of a 'unified syncretism,' the cultural multiplicity, which Carpentier assumed to the foundation of a 'marvelous reality' and its syncretism, proves to be an uncontrolled polysemy, a baroque heterotopia whose weave, whose macula, cannot integrate the sundry threads, cannot synthesize its variability into transcendent unity'" (101). Lois Parkinson Zamora describes the baroque as "a model of a dynamic, decentered, and inclusive . . . perspective such as is necessary to understand and express New World realities" (101).[7]

As an aesthetic practice that multiplies, proliferates, reverses, and fragments the singularity of origins, the baroque is also understood as a rethinking and realignment of gender and race as categories marking difference. From the smallest grammatical unit to the narrative as a whole, Carpentier's baroque prose jumps through and between different linguistic temporalities, tense switches, anachronistic vocabularies, extended epic time frames and the like, never staying firmly enough within a cultural matrix to constitute or construct a stylistic integrity. For Carpentier, the existence of ancient forms in contemporary times, the present presence of the archaic, disturbs the linearity of narrative:

> The Latin American of today, who lives with the illiterate masses—the literacy rate has reached, in the great island of the Caribbean, the scandalous number of ninety per cent . . .—lives with the masses which correspond culturally with that of medieval Europe. . . . Before this presence of the past in the future, living in a today where already can be seen palpitations of the future, the Latin American novelist has to break the rules of traditional temporality in the narrative in order to invent what best converges with the material treated, or make use of—one takes the techniques where one finds them—others which adjust themselves to the focuses of reality. ("Problemática del tiempo y el idioma en la moderna novela latinoamericana" [1975] (1990), 215)

The shifting locations of historical time, marked by different racial populations, recalls a recapitulatory logic where racial difference signifies temporal schisms, thus distorting chronologies and lineages. "The illiterate Caribbean masses" can only be understood as blacks, mulattos, and the indigenous. Interrelated with the chronologies of race, the other factor marking time here is, of course, the different levels of technological assimilation and, in particular, the different levels of mass media saturation. Racial difference itself seems to be read, in fact, as a degree of mass literacy. As Carpentier once said, "America is the only continent where different ages coexist, where a man from the twentieth century can shake hands with another from the fourth or with another population without newspapers or communications, a population which resembles that of the Middle Ages or exists contemporarily with another from a province closer to the

Romanticism of 1850 than to today's epoque. Going up the Orinoco is like going back in time" (see Romeu, 325).

The baroque, says González Echevarría, is foremost and essentially a problem of reproduction. "A mistress of love," he writes of Fernando de Roja's 1499 work *Celestina,* which, he argues, inaugurates the genre: "Celestina is hardly the agent of social restoration and continuity. She is the enabler in a commerce of bodies, desires, and reputations that is the opposite and sometimes the parody of the rituals through which society renews itself: courtship and marriage. Celestina's brew works against the brood" (1993: 10). For Carpentier, virginity frames the borders of the baroque, and mothering configures its modes of reproduction. In "Lo barroco y lo real maravilloso," Carpentier claims that the baroque is a "horror of emptiness" (172), a creative pressure that "appears to break the frame which surrounds it," (173) and that results in a splitting or proliferating from the center. The contemporary Cuban novelist Severo Sarduy reworks Carpentier's baroque, a racial difference marked by a recapitulatory fragmentation of time, into a Lacanian, poststructuralist narrative of sexual difference in the symbolic. The absence and the inevitability of the historical referent—in Carpentier's case, the simultaneous opacity and transparency of colonialism as origin—is also, as Sarduy claims, in the baroque, a primary subjective fragmentation. For Sarduy, the baroque is a reflection of other forms, of new and separate emergences, but a reflection that nevertheless breaks away from its own image. Borrowing from Roland Barthes' Lacanian theories of *jouissance,* Sarduy defines the baroque as a displacement of the image, a reproduction of an empty center, an absent origin, and the desire for that origin: "The present baroque, the neobaroque, reflects structurally the disharmony, the rupture of homogeneity, of the logos as absolute, the lack which constitutes our fundamental episteme . . . , a desire which can not reach its object, desire for which the logos has not organized more than a screen which hides its lack . . . the partial object has become the lost object" (103). Undermining the status that privileges the logos as the primary and singular signifier of difference, the baroque, according to Sarduy, represents the impossibility of reproduction, the desire for the inaccessible object.

In *The Lost Steps,* the narrator-protagonist's voyage into the jungle is the enactment of a desire for an origin that, in the end, is inaccessible. The sign marking the entrance into the jungle, that is, into the primitive, represents an abstract and eternal design, a crypt, a reproduction of the narrator-protagonist's own conception: "But there was a sign cut in its bark, three V's, one fitting vertically into another in a design that might have been repeated ad infinitum, but which here was multiplied only in the reflection of the waters" (159). One day later the boat hits a storm. As the waters lurch into the canoe from bow to stern, as the boat founders in semi-submersion, the narrator-protagonist seeks refuge and salvation in Rosario's embrace, regressing to infancy: "My reason gone, unable to control my fear, I clung to Rosario, seeking the warmth of her body, no longer as a lover, but like a child clinging to its mother's neck.... Rosario, her teeth clenched, protecting my head as though it were that of her newborn babe in a moment of danger, displayed an amazing fortitude" (170). In a sense, the narrator-protagonist's entrance into the jungle happens as his own recapitulation of historical time; the border opening into the jungle is the birth canal through which he must pass, the mother's body serving as an environmental obstacle, a prohibition against entering providing the only path of entry: "The boats could hardly keep afloat as we moved from eddy to eddy, nosing through the gorges, riding over boulders, tacking quickly to skirt a rapid, always on the verge of capsizing, surrounded by foam, in tortured boards that groaned the length of the keel" (170).[8] The opening of the birth canal gives passage into another culture, another race that is secret and inaccessible.

As race and recapitulation recreate the woman's body as a figure of inaccessibility—a crypt—images of obstructed birth and failing motherhood are mapped onto the central problems of (oppositional) subjectivity that the text explores. In fact, *The Lost Steps* is, from the beginning, a chronicle of the narrator-protagonist's discontinuity within his subjective tale and his search for self-integration. The unknowability of the self—the impossibility of the self-birth of the artist—is throughout the narrative linked to female infertility—first to European artistic sterility and then to the limited reproduction of interracial breeding. "Within me," he comes to conclude, "another stirred who was also I, and who did not quite fit his own image; he and I were uncomfortably superimposed on one another, like plates handled by an apprentice lithographer in which the yellows and the reds do not completely coincide" (234). The split in subjectivity—the nonconformity of language to itself which the baroque manifests—is here constituted through the inaccessibility of an autobiographical enunciation, of origin.

Perhaps the source of this division, and the desire for its erasure, reside in the very idea of an "autobiographical novel," a fiction that is real and not real. The problem arises, as many critics have remarked,[9] in the first sentence: "Four years and seven months had passed since I had seen the white-pillared house, with the austere pediment that gave it the severity of a courthouse; now, among the furniture and decorations, whose positions never varied, I had the distressing sensation that time had turned back" (3). In the Spanish, the sentence is in the imperfect tense, which is the same for both first- and third-person enunciations. It is impossible to tell here, therefore, whether the narrative is speaking from the first person or the third, given the repetition of the imperfect tense and the absence of any marking pronouns. In addition, the sentence makes that very use of the imperfect tense ambiguous, as the tenses of the verbs are jarred by the adverbial intervention "ahora." The sentence resides simultaneously in an undefined historical moment, a moment of historical repetition, and the unqualified, expanding present. Meanwhile, the narrator is telling of a return or a repetition that never happens and whose possibility is negated. The very difficulty of uttering "I," of situating or insinuating an integrated subject—of being born—is part of the structure of the sentence itself, which divides and combines the "auto" of the biography into the present and the ever-returning, repeating, recapitulating, inaccessible past.

The play between fiction and nonfiction, which the very genre "autobiographical novel" presupposes, is therefore grounded in the uprootedness of speaking the "I" that would claim it as real, as autobiography, but uncertainly so. According to González Echevarría (1977), Carpentier was complicit in creating a critical uncertainty about his own life (31). His public declarations and journalistic writings insisted that the text of *The Lost Steps* actually came to him suddenly while he was traveling the Orinoco, and that the characters are based on the people he met there. González Echevarría finds contradictions in these accounts and calls Carpentier's own investment in making the text autobiographical through fiction an "invocation of the empirical author" (22).

The novel itself echoes the idea that autobiography is fiction. The scene of the narrator's birth at the cryptic entrance to the jungle presages the birth of the endangered utterance of the "I" that would govern autobiography as a Latin American literature of difference, that is, as the "real." The novel begins with an exploration of inauthenticity, of fiction, playing on the instability of the line differentiating the falsity of Western art from the "real" of difference. The narrator-protagonist walks onto a theatrical stage; the architectural features in the first sentence cited above are actually, the text only later reveals, props on that stage. The play has been enacted every day for the past four years and seven months. In each presentation, Ruth, the narrator-protagonist's wife, has recited her role, receding into automated repetition. The reference of "four years and seven months" is to President Lincoln's Gettysburg Address and, through that, to the U.S. color line, which blocks the birth of the real. Ruth's indefatigable and sterile repetition has seeped into every aspect of their conjugal life, as even their sex is performed according to a fixed time schedule, by which they faithfully replicate the act at the same time every Sunday. When Ruth does get pregnant, it is only as a media simulation, a fake, a melodramatic play-acting put on for sensationalistic reporting, sentimentalism, and flash.

The eternal, infernal, and sterile repetition obfuscates the birth of the subject, the autobiographical gesture, a progression governed by a desire to tell the origin, to reach the source, in reproduction:

> There were gaps of weeks in the chronicle [*crónica*] of my existence, seasons that left with me no real memory, no unusual sensation, no enduring emotion; days when every gesture left me with the obsession that I had done the same thing before under identical circumstances—that I had been sitting in the same corner, that I had been telling the same story. . . . When my birthday was celebrated among the same faces, in the same places, with the same song sung in chorus, the thought invariably struck me that the only difference between my previous birthday and this one was the extra candle on the cake, which tasted exactly like the last one. (9)

The choice of the word *crónica* would bring the histories of conquest into play, as though the telling of the life of the self would coincide with or recapitulate the telling of the life of the continent originating in tales of rape and conquest. The birth of narrative is, then, intertwined with the obstructed birth of the autobiographical subject as difference, an obstruction linked to a colonial history of forced interracial sex.

The obstructed birth of autobiography is further reflected in the narrator-protagonist's constantly deferred baptism, where his name cannot be uttered until Rosario names him and still is never present in the text. "That day for the first time Rosario called me by my name, repeating it again and again, as though its syllables had to be molded anew, and in her mouth it took on a sonority so strange, so unexpected, that I was spellbound by the word I knew best when I heard it as though it had just been created" (157). Here, the act of naming, of baptism, is complicated not only by the use of the past subjunctive, which introduces doubt and uncertainty, but also by the fact that the text refuses to utter the name, refuses to reproduce the word that Rosario, ironically, repeats silently but repeats as new.

The idea that autobiography, especially when linked to expressions of racial, gender, or "multicultural" experience, is necessarily an oppositional category, a practice of resistance, a self-defining or revolutionary situation of empowerment, or a challenge to hegemonic oppressions and silencings, has recently become a contentious issue within postcolonial debates. With *The Lost Steps*, Carpentier does not easily fall into a tradition of oppositional nationalisms that would come to fashion themselves into a postcolonial configuration of meanings, symbols, relationships, and interests in the wake of mostly African and Asian movements of decolonization in the 1960s. In terms of Latin American histories, this novel, published more than one hundred years after the wars of independence by a Cuban national educated in France and residing in Venezuela, is hardly an expression of a struggle against imperial or monistic power,[10] or a formative crystallization of subjective agency as a mode of resistance, or foundation for self-governance and autonomy. J. Jorge Klor de Alva has, indeed, argued that Latin America is not a valid representative of the postcolonial condition because, he says, the history of the independence movements places these regions within a tradition of liberalism rather than in the radical nationalistic agendas, violent battles for political recognition of the margins, and struggles for identity found within late twentieth-century postcolonial movements. According to Klor de Alva, in the absence of cohesion among the governing classes in Latin America, a discourse of *mestizaje*, "a euphemism for the overwhelming presence of Western influences" (250), developed in order to mobilize a discrete regionalism, based on indigenous emblems, around which to formulate operational identities for international negotiations in the postindependence period. Meanwhile, colonial-like relations were still maintained between the elites in the center and the indigenous populations on the margins.

Nevertheless, the negotiations Carpentier performs—of continental difference through autobiographical inscriptions of racial identities and colonial fantasies—developed into a "magic realist" literary form. That form provided, in turn, one of the conceptual frameworks underpinning postcolonial narratives and theories. In Carpentier's novel, the unnameable proliferation of life forms names the margins as the referent for agency, autonomy, and identity. Within the novel's logic, liberation is articulated from the margins. Is there an alternative way of considering identity besides always thinking of it as either essential and immobilizing but perhaps useful for political cohesion and alliance or, rather, constructable and therefore deconstructable? Is there a way, possibly, of reinserting economic considerations and questions of equity into models that posit the political and linguistic variability of identity? Is there a sense, indeed, in which the kind of hybrid identities developed by Carpentier and then appropriated into new postcolonial scholarship has allowed for the obfuscation of the economy, masking the politics of hardship by romanticizing the authenticity of the margins?

Within the postcolonial theoretical debates, the politics of identity—with its representations of subjective wholeness, its essentialisms of the self and its overdetermined marginalities—is pitted against a more self-professedly radical (because more deconstructive) approach to identity. According to Ashcroft, Griffiths, and Triffin in their groundbreaking work *The Empire Writes Back*, postcolonial literature posits the inadequacy of Western hegemony for fairly and faithfully representing the "experience" (2), frequently "race-based" (15), of the colonized outside of the imperial center.[11] Within such theories of postcolonial literatures, race becomes a sign of referential rootedness and transparency that solidifies the autobiographical utterance as a form of representativity, a certainty of knowledge to be stated or performed in the face of silencing oppressions.

However, in *The Lost Steps*, racial identities are constantly destabilized, providing paradigms of illegitimacy, illegibility, and more mobile conscriptions of self within political strategies. A postcolonial deconstructive critique of autobiography, by mobilizing figures of race, would call into question the metaphysics of realism by fragmenting the narrative cohesion and rational consistency of the speaking "I" and by uprooting its referential logics. Sara Suleri, in her essay "Woman Skin Deep: Feminism and the Postcolonial Condition," criticizes the autobiographical gestures prevalent and even occasionally imperative in much current postcolonial and feminist theoretical work; for example, the "articulation of marginality," the objectification of "lived experience" (252), and the "will to subjectivity" (247), as "a low-grade romanticism" (248) and a return to the bourgeois project of realism. Gayatri Spivak, as well, has argued that speaking from the position of a Third World subject "gets bogged down in ... homogenization" (63), creating reified representations of ethnic identities that, in their determining singularity and authentication of knowledge, produce new enclaves of silence. "There are many subject positions which one must inhabit," she writes. "One is not just one thing.... In fact, for the person who does the 'speaking as' something, it is a problem of distancing from one's self, whatever that self might be" (60). Just as in Carpentier's fictions, which defer the autobiographical, the speaking postcolonial subject in these theories is inaccessible, indeterminable, unknowable, both reproducing the real and transforming it.

In these debates over identity in postcolonial thought, taking an oppositional position depends upon whether the name is recognized or disallows recognition. The politics of recognition, however, seems concerned with an aesthetic orientation toward different rituals, customs, and life practices, and so obscures the way that both recognition and nonrecognition maintain uneven distributions of economic and political power. For Carpentier, hybridity seems to dissolve the name and its identity, which then need to be reconstituted, but reconstituting the name does not coincide with new economic relations. The narrator-protagonist can access new cultures in the jungle and feel revitalized in the knowledge of the new aesthetic they offer. The metropolis where the narrator-protagonist returns to still controls the means of production and the distribution channels that allow him to secure the raw energy of primitive production for his own profit, career advancement, and artistic sensibility. By defining interracial, postcolonial relations as the desire for difference and newness, Alejo Carpentier is concealing the economic relations that allow indigenous cultures to be valued and named as commodities, even as indigenous peoples are exploited as a cheap industrial labor force or become casualties in the cross-fire between international drug rings and neoliberal power brokers. To posit postcolonial subjectivity as oppositional, not only does there need to be a recognition of different experiences but also an accompanying leveling of economic power between nations and populations.

The images of obstructed birth in *The Lost Steps*, are produced in part through referencing the color line with its politics of sexuality. Interracial sterility is invoked as defining the cultural border between the United States and its Latin American Other. For example, the play in which Ruth is employed is a play about Lincoln. The pillars mentioned in the first sentence represent the entrance to a southern plantation. The allusion to the U.S. color line helps to situate the banality and sterility of this false cosmopolitan culture in the permanence and repetition of historical racial divisions, the absence of a love that would create the new and give birth to the subject of art. The artificiality of the theater is produced by the U.S. taboo against racial mixing.

"Lo real," on the other hand, the capacitation of the authentic autobiographical subject as Latin American *mestizo*, would break the mimetic cycle of theatrical performance, of inauthenticity, situated in racial/sexual segregation. Critics have well documented the way the time indications in the presentation of the novel as diary become, through the course of the text, gradually less firmly schematized in the repetition of Mondays at the beginning of the work week. Halfway through the novel (the first subchapter of chapter 3), the dates heading the entries become less stringent, as time seems to escape from the confinements of a weekly reversion to the same. The third subchapter of chapter 3 reinscribes the dating sequence, but in error. Marked "Tuesday, the 12th," the entry skips over the Monday on which the twelfth would fall according to the novel's own temporal logic. The error, the break from repetition, occurs when the narrator-protagonist and, therefore, the text itself has crossed into the jungle, leaving behind the theater of the color line with its racial separatism, its antiprogressive circularities, its impossible reproductions, its clock rhythms, and its constant recursions to the same.

The border between the city and the jungle—the colonial border—is meant to coincide, then, with the border between the inauthentic repetitions of the U.S. city and "lo real," the authenticity of the Latin American jungle in biodiverse transformation. However, this demarcating separation is constantly undermined. The continual statement of the difference between the two settings becomes, like the first- and third-person subjective divisions and the tense markers in the first sentence, like the site of a southern plantation and its falsification on a theatrical set, the very site of their confluence. Much of this dubiousness of placement, where what is identical suddenly becomes a radical difference, is treated as an ambiguity of legacy in which Latin America is seen as embedded in Western literary traditions as much as it is different. As González Echevarría remarks, "Instead of the unmediated presence that Carpentier seeks in his voyage to the source of time and history, he finds that road to paradise littered with texts that form an unpliable and dense memory from which he can find no release. He is caught in the paradox of being 'in the entrails of virginal America,' the fruit of a fatherless, unmediated conception; the product of an originality which denies anteriority while affirming at every step that his own text is a repetition—a new version, perhaps whose lineage can be traced" (1977, 174). Indeed, the narrator-protagonist's steps into the jungle are steps backward through the history of texts, as his resolution to compose the most original choral work by setting the *Odyssey* to music suggests. González Echevarría (1997) has said that the textualization of the Latin American landscape in *The Lost Steps* is a sign that Latin American literature has always been firmly embedded within the Western tradition of modern literature: "This foundational element, this burning proximity to the origins of the modern tradition, is what distinguishes Latin American literature, what makes it different and hence capable of being compared with other literatures of the West. The question is how Latin American literature reads that tradition, how it incorporates it and incorporates itself within it" (56). The title of the novel is actually a distorted reflection of Proust's *A la recherche du temps perdu*. In fact, the act of remembrance, which structures both the narrative and the journey back through cultural, historical, biological, and personal time, is modeled on a Proustian *mémoire involuntaire*. The narrator-protagonist, hearing Beethoven's *Ninth Symphony* in the jungle, is overtaken by a memory of his father. The memory is of his father's nostalgia for the Old World, which inspires the narrator to travel to Europe. Arriving, the narrator finds only a Europe in ruins, a decadent and cruel and culturally bankrupt Europe, riddled with the horror of concentration camps, on the eve of World War II. González Echevarría (1977) attributes this passage to the influence of Spengler, whose notion of the cyclical rise and fall of civilizations was attractive to Carpentier for his privileging of America as the peak of a new avant-garde. The repetition of Proust's title in Carpentier's "original" work is illustrative of Carpentier's Spenglerian belief that every rise of civilization follows the same cyclical trajectory but in a different place.

The place that both differentiates the city from the jungle and conflates them, where Western tradition both merges with and separates from the cultures of Carpentier's "América," is textualized through the body of the hybrid woman. Though "the thousand books I had read" (107) are what separate the narrator-protagonist from Rosario, he still sees Rosario's body itself as textualized in those books already read: "Rosario . . . was like a St. Cecilia or St. Lucy. . . . Relationships became established between her flesh and the ground we were trading, relationships proclaimed by sun-darkened skins" (106–7). In fact, the very biology of racial mixing in Rosario is a reproduction of a European origin in Greece, where literature was born: "This traveler of the wastelands and the fog was of no more mixed origins than the races that for centuries had come together in the melting-pot of the Mediterranean" (81). In the end, the jungle itself becomes the inauthentic, the citational, reinforcing the narrator-protagonist's uncanny feeling of never having departed the farther away he goes, "the strange sensation of not having traveled, of always having been *there*" (58).

Yet, this very uncanny repetition—what makes the jungle into a mere reflection of the world of the city—is, at the very same time, what makes it different: "What amazed me most was the inexhaustible mimetism of virgin nature. Everything here seemed something else, thus creating a world of appearances that concealed reality, casting doubt on many truths" (165). Like Rosario's repetition of the narrator's name, evolutionary repetition of the same becomes in the jungle paradoxically something "new." The "new" is here reproduced through the inaccessibility—the unknowability—of a nature that, as virgin, has not yet been named. What follows is a list of species; being transformations of nature, these species fall outside any attempt at signification. Ironically, the animals resist their taxonomical names. They are different and signify differently, because the jungle, repeating their forms, transforms them: "The vines seemed snakes.... The world of the lizard-cucumber, the chestnut-hedgehog, the cocoon-centipede, the carrot-larva, the electric fish that electrocutes from the dregs of the slime" (165–66). Interspecies crossing, with its reproductive proliferation of natural hybrid differences, becomes, like the narrator-protagonist's desire for Rosario, the concept through which a Latin American artistic subjectivity can be produced as different, in its *mestizaje*, from the cultural sterility of the metropolis.

This theme of locating difference—the escape from and repetition of the same—in the autobiographical enunciation might provide an opening for thinking through *The Lost Steps* in terms of some recent theoretical interrogations of postcolonial studies. Basically, Carpentier chronicles the emergence of subjectivity and creative agency by (1) narrating it through a colonial historicity, and (2) environmentally localizing it through the difficult naming of its nature and geographies, to make it specifically Latin American. Carpentier is here employing biological figures to reformulate rhetorical gestures in which Latin American *mestizaje* would develop—as Retamar, echoing José Martí, would say in *Calibán*—into a symbol for "a vast zone for which mestizaje is not an accident [as it was, for Retamar, in Africa and Asia], but the essence, the central line: us, our mestizo America" (9). Carpentier provides a way of imagining the subject of resistance as it is mapped through stories of subjugation in colonial conquest and rape. Such figures of resistance are later picked up by postcolonial writings as a political-discursive strategy, a model for agency.

Indeed, similar to the ways in which Carpentier revises modernist aesthetics by narrating "the new" as the history of hybridity in rape, some postcolonial perspectives have placed hybridity as a central thematic in their theoretical investigations. Within postcolonial writings, hybridity calls into question the legacy of traditions. Ideas such as sovereignty and autonomy, regionalism and nationalism, individualism and universalism, are borrowed from foreign places and claimed as local realities. Particularly, within Latin American studies, the current grappling with the theoretical insights of new postcolonial thinking has tended to hark back toward the almost mythologized origins of modern Latin American nationalisms in order to uphold Latin America as a privileged site of hybrid resistance to hegemonic cultures. For instance, speaking of the vast urban migrations that have transformed Latin American cities during the course of the twentieth century into spaces of multicultural complexity, Antonio Cornejo-Polar has developed a theory of heterogeneity that focuses on Latin American empiricism, with its evidence of racial mixing, as the core of postcolonial literary potential:

> I suspect that the contents of multiplicity, instability and displacement which [the category of migration] carries with it implicitly, and its inexcusable reference to a dispersed variety of socio-cultural spaces which spread out as much as they are articulated through migration itself, make it an especially appropriate category for the study of the intense heterogeneity of a good part of Latin American literature. Of course: the magnitude of the phenomenon of rural to urban migration also appears to endorse, from the level of empiricism if you like, its hermeneutic aptitude. (838)

Through a circular yet paradoxical movement, Latin American postcolonial thinking has tried to find a place in universalized metropolitan academic discourses by making literary constructions of its own specific histories; the importing of Western theory can be justified because it specifically describes the contemporary social realities of Latin America and therefore is more true there. By restating the theory of postcolonial hybridity as Latin American empirical reality, such theory, like Carpentier's aesthetics, repeats the name and terminology of a Western dominant discourse as something "new," an "American" difference.

What such theories of hybridity neglect, however, is that migrancy is not a fluffy abstraction challenging, on the level of contending fictions, economic rationality with its regulations of people, places, and identities. Rather, urbanization is a very real result of the very real imbalances caused by a very real capitalist globalization and, in turn, causing very real human suffering all over the world, and linguistic indeterminacy or representational ambiguity had done little to change things. Like Carpentier, Latin American postcolonial studies have reified colonization, conquest, and their aftermath into an aesthetic category constructing Latin America as "the real," a metaphoric potential for speaking an "American" empirical difference as a challenge to, and repetition of, fields of knowledge produced as universal. The use of colonization and conquest as symbols of national difference has tended to empty the content of the actual historical event, to remove the actual practice of genocide, as well as absenting the very real victims of its current reoccurrences, the crushing of marginal populations and popular political resistance under the weight of global power. As Hernán Vidal, for example, writes, "Cycles of renewal of Latin American literary criticism [are] initiated based not on the problems of the cultures being studied but rather on the new critical theories periodically introduced into the publishing market" (115). And Román de la Campa adds, "But one would have to ask if this whole critical program [of postcolonialism] does not respond mostly to the cultural needs and the academic market which emanate from the United States and Europe" (1996: 715). What Carpentier's work contributes to the current theoretical interchange, then, is a demonstration of the discursive process through which Latin America becomes the referent and base-line "truth" born of yet another Western theory of cultural fragmentation.

This is not to say that Latin America should be made into the "real" in just another empirical site; that is, as the "real" of genocide, capitalist, and media domination, instead of the "real" of migrant urbanity, the "real" that would break open the borders of identity, reconceptualizing the disparities between the eternal essence and its repetitions in fiction. Rather, what is needed is a careful analysis of how the market and the media are shaping the way people live, making some modes of life untenable while forcing mass movements to other spaces. In fact, some postcolonial theory has considered market expansion central to any analysis of modern culture. Stuart Hall, for example, has argued that the postcolonial, instead of periodizing all histories through references to Western incursions and withdrawals, takes into account the vast reconfiguration of the globe implemented through a colonial history whose ramifications were felt everywhere: "By 'colonisation', the 'post-colonial' references something more than direct rule over certain areas of the world by the imperial powers. I think it is signifying the whole process of expansion, exploration, conquest, colonisation and imperial hegemonisation which constituted the 'outer face,' the constitutive outside, of European and then Western capitalist modernity after 1492" (249). In other words, the movement of capital on a global scale must be central to any consideration of cultural representation and its politics.

The narrator-protagonist of *The Lost Steps* plans to turn the lives of the primitive peoples he encounters in the jungle into a musical score in the narrative line of the *Odyssey,* to be performed in music halls in cities across Europe. The narrator-protagonist's thrill of appropriation—his own thirst to stage the culture of the jungle as a universally broadcasted media spectacle, to commodify it in order to create a new aesthetics of culture—ends in the disappearance of the jungle cultures from the world stage. Even as the text suggests that Rosario and her community have hidden themselves away from the West and its composers on their own initiative, one can only wonder, given the current incursions of capital in the jungle, if their disappearance did not amount to a more substantial erasure: the possibility that they were or would be totally wiped out. The idea of "disappearance" in Latin America ("estar desaparecido") has just such a history. In postcolonial theory, the use of Latin American discourses of hybridity as a sign of liberation can indeed serve as hypocritical masks to hegemonic domination and genocidal practices. As Klor de Alva points out, "The culmination of colonialism was the disappearance of the indigenes and their world, *not into a brew of Indian-Spanish composition, but into the cultural vortex of the West*" (1992: 6; original emphasis).

In *The Lost Steps,* colonialism becomes the term by which the difference of the speaking subject gets posited, as well as the statement of difference exposed as fallacious, fictional, impossible, and inaccessible. What is more, Carpentier evokes colonial history as a signifier of difference by constructing femininity as a colonial space. Rosario, as a figure of the racial hybridities brought into play through colonial contact, becomes a sign for the essentialized identity as well as the instabilities and incoherencies of difference that is the Latin American subject. Rosario's various positions in Carpentier's novel serve to create a fissure through that the narrator-protagonist must journey in order to access "lo real," the "new" in art that corresponds to the difference of Latin American identity, its landscapes of interbreeding hybridities. "My formations, her prejudices," ruminates the narrator-protagonist, "all that she had been taught, all that she valued, at that moment seemed to me irreconcilable factors. I kept telling myself that none of all this had any bearing on the ever-possible coupling of the body of a man and a woman, and yet I knew that an entire culture . . . separated me from that forehead" (107). As the pivot around which realism, subjectivity, and autobiographical presence get simultaneously articulated and undermined, the narrator-protagonist's desire for Rosario produces a geographical border, a spatial and temporal rupture through which Latin American difference can begin to be described.

Like the *vanguardista* intellectuals of the time, the narrator-protagonist recreates colonial relations, but his sexual relations with Rosario represent his power. Giovannini considers that the project of *The Lost Steps* resides in "the wish . . . to arrive at a synthesis of European aesthetics with the virgin 'reality' of Latin America" or "a possible fusion between Art and Nature" (159). Indeed, the narrator-protagonist's access to mass media allows him to appropriate the culture of the jungle for his own artistic rejuvenation, just as his sex life is made to live again in his passion for Rosario, his sexual dominance over her. "There the woman 'serves' the man in the noblest sense of the word, creating the home with every gesture" (154). The narrator-protagonist's decision to leave the jungle is predicated, in part, upon his need for his composition to be sold and even performed in the metropolis: "A score that is not played is utterly valueless. A work of art is meant for others—above all, music, which by its very nature can reach vast audiences" (225). Whatever the narrator-protagonist means here by "vast audiences," it is certainly not the people in his immediate vicinity, the people of the jungle. The narrator realizes that the music he is composing would not be of interest to the people of Santa Mónica, who are still making music as though in a medieval age, the age of performance, of the immediate presence of audience. The main difference the narrator-protagonist remarks between his own composition and the music played in the jungle is that his is and must be written, as *crónica,* something which El Adelantado and the others do not comprehend because they compose as they perform, believing that a gift of a guitar should be sufficient to the production of music, that paper is not necessary (280–81). The narrator-protagonist himself points out the absurdity of his mission to compose for an audience which he, at the same time, has renounced:

> Rosario asked me to whom I was writing letters, inasmuch as there was no post office there. This mistake, the vision of a letter meant to travel, but which could not, suddenly made me aware of the vanity of everything I had been doing since the day before. . . . I had chosen the moment of my escape

> from the places where a work of mine could be heard to begin really to compose. It was foolish, absurd, laughable. (225)

Santiago Colás discusses the Cuban *vanguardista* intellectual and the subsequent "Boom" generation writers who latched onto the Cuban cause as constructing a gulf, an imbalance, between themselves and the masses by employing innovation and technique in order to sell their productions to Western audiences: "The Boom writers' self-conscious anti-imperialist declaration of achieved revolutionary independence [in the trademark of 'magical realism'] was underwritten by a material dependency facilitated by their re-creation of a colonial relations with their own people" (391). Clearly, in Carpentier's case, the immediacy, the sensation the jungle offers through Rosario's submissive sexuality is the raw product to be wrapped up in an aesthetic consciousness, dominated as it enters global commercial circulation as an orchestral jingle. Colonial history, along with its present legacy of unequal power relations, is commodified through its eroticization.

If the naming of the monstrous new forms of species crossing in the jungle, the colonial act of domination and possession *par excellence*, represents a potential consummation, then Mouche's activities with the Canadian painter would resist the name. Indeed, the narrator calls them variably "a kind of chill indifference toward everything, a new self-sufficiency" (70), "the most hideous physical possibilities" (70), "the greatest physical perfidies" (63), "copulations that left no memory" (63), "suspicious attentions" (125), and finally, "an offense which ... is worse than the worst epithet, worse than insulting the mother, worse than being driven from home, worse than spitting in the face of the nearest and dearest, worse than questioning their marital fidelity, worse than calling them bitches, whores" (149). In fact, what Mouche does with women—her abomination—is precisely figured out of the text, blocking reproductions of "lo real." Obstructing the inscription of "la huella" (the footprint, the impression, the trace), the desire to create the impression of the exceptional by telling the autobiographical (72), the affair with the Canadian painter is never more than what the narrator-protagonist's imagination conjures up, what he suspects. Her later sexual assault on Rosario is an inference, a wordless reflection, happening in an inaccessible place where the narration cannot go.

The space of incomprehensibility and unreproducibleness that Mouche's act marks in the text becomes a sign of a vital and violent separation, a non-communicability between the simulated life of the city and the living sensuality of the jungle. Rosario is the cipher through which the culture of the "new" would be reproduced, whereas Mouche is the vital connection to the world of *allá*, which suspends cohabitation and mixing with the forestial forms. In her propensities to lesbian acts, Mouche is the automated reproduction of European avant-garde formulaics in surrealism's "the unusual." In her lesbianism, she is the prohibition of the birth of "the new" as a culture or a literature of Latin American national difference and separate origins. Through contrast to Mouche's sterility, Rosario's infertility gets framed as leading to something else: a just resolution in the expectation of reproduction. As Lourdes Rojas-Paiewonsky states, "Next to the strong image of Rosario, heroine in defense of her heterosexuality, the image of Mouche is a clear stamp of failure, of the anti-natural (her lesbianism), of the foreign" (133). The narrator-protagonist, in fact, is constantly pointing out Mouche's failures at assimilation in the jungle world, with its hybrid reproductions, metamorphosis, and symbiosis: "Mouche in this environment was an absurd being, torn from a future where the forest had been replaced by the avenue. She belonged to another age, another epoch" (149).

Mouche's inability to separate from her identification with the city makes her body a site of deterioration and inauthenticity. The cosmetics she needs to maintain her "natural beauty" and theatrics now unobtainable, her appearance loses its attraction, and she becomes susceptible to diseases:

> What surprised me now was that the very substance of her body, the flesh of which it was made, seemed to have faded since the morning of that last day of navigation. Her skin, roughened by the hard water, had reddened, revealing areas of coarse pores around her nose and temples. Her hair had taken on the look of tow, greenish-blond in color, streaky, making evident how much its normal coppery hue owed to the careful use of tints. Under her blouse, stained by strange oils that dripped from the sails, her breasts seemed less firm, and the polish peeled off nails broken. (122)

Every aspect of her physicality seems artificial, as underneath the coverings of her make-up and hair dyes, her body seems wasted, undone. Through

Mouche, the narrator-protagonist is able to construct a criticism of the market economy that he has, though ambiguously, renounced, a vision of a consumerism that in its nonreproductiveness is sickly and sterile, unfaithful and empty, beneath its appearances. Mouche's sexuality positions her as representing a desire destructive to the fecundity of "lo real," the interaction between local expression and a wider global penetration.

The parasitical sickness that invades, takes over, and eats away at Mouche's body, symbolically linked to European modernism, is what both separates the narrator-protagonist from Rosario and what joins him to her. Coming in between the lovers in their first act of lovemaking, Mouche's malaria-ravaged face becomes the signifier of their difference, the border between their bodies overcome (momentarily):

> But even as we sought a better position, a faint, hoarse voice was spitting insults in our ears, startling us apart. We had rolled under the hammock, oblivious of the presence of the owner of the voice. And Mouche's head was hanging over us, her mouth twisted, sneering, slavering, her tangled hair falling over her forehead, giving her a Medusa look.... Soon the voice above us wandered off in the ravings of delirium. The disjoined bodies found each other once more, and between my face and the death-mask face of Mouche, hanging from the hammock, with one arm trailing limp, Rosario's heavy hair fell like a curtain. She rested her elbows on the floor to impose her rhythm upon me. (152)

Mouche's face, disappearing beyond recognition, becomes the Medusa head, the demoniacal expression, in psychoanalysis, of the little boy's acknowledgment of his mother's difference, the threat of castration. The narrator-protagonist's rejection of Mouche serves the absolute merging between Rosario as raw cultural expression and the logic of her reproduction, her ability to circulate as a sign of the cultural fecundity of the global market.

"My escape has been consummated," claims the narrator-protagonist. The narrator-protagonist's voyage into the jungle, his desire for a colonial origin, is treated as a marriage. If the consummation would occur, the narrator-protagonist's marriage to the jungle would consist of naming, of naming the virgin forest, vegetational forms that have never yet been named. Naming would be a type of penetration, entering the crypt, reading the cipher.

The virgin (forest) is without name: "Leaning over the devil's caldron," says the narrator-protagonist, "I felt the vertigo of space. I knew that if I let myself come under the spell of what I was looking upon here, this prenatal world, I would end up by hurling myself down, burying myself in this fearful density of leaves which would one day disappear from the planet without having been given a name, without having been re-created by the Word" (206). To give the virgin (forest) a name, to consummate a relation with it, would presage the (im)possible birth of "lo real" as an original hybridity, a colonial cross of cultures, an item of pure erotic sensation aestheticized and commodified as the global market.

The references to the "virgin forest" and the need to penetrate it through naming suggest that colonization is here insinuated through a metaphorics of masculinity. Indeed, the very artificiality of the city, with its false columns, its semblances of façades, its theaters, its banality of reproduction and repetition, diminishes masculinities, making them impotent by preventing consummation with its naming of the "new." "How hard it is," contemplates the narrator-protagonist about his life in the city, "to become a man again when one has ceased to be a man" (22). The primitive, its environments and its presence in "lo real," promise a return to a primal culture of masculinity.[12] Realizing his resemblance to primitive man with his outstanding virility, the narrator-protagonist revitalizes his masculine potency, his ability to create and to name the "new," through desiring the primitive in women. In the crossing of the color line, in the consummation with the forest, men, says the narrator-protagonist, become more manly: "A mysterious solidarity was established between the animal with well-hung testicles which covered its female deeper than any other and man [in the Lands of the Horse]" (114). This hypersexualization (and racialization) of the male organ, as a sign of universal humanity in primitive desire, becomes the source, infers the narrator-protagonist, of a will to pleasure in conquest and miscegenation, his first copulation with Rosario: "I had sown myself beneath the down I stroked with the hand of the master, and my gesture closed the cycle of a joyful commingling of bloods that have met" (153). Desire and pleasure here take the place of military and corporate force in crossing borders between nations and cultures.

The narrative, however, never reaches the expected romantic resolution in marriage. The mobilization of legal and economic interests, acquisitions and alliances that would come into play through marriage are deferred by, it seems at first, the narrator-protagonist's previous marriage to Ruth. But the text eventually subordinates this rationale as an excuse, a deceit, a protocol that could be overcome in legal battles and bureaucratic chores. Ultimately, Rosario refuses marriage. Marriage for her means, she says, that she would be subject to men's undue excesses and abuses of drink and deceit without recourse to the one defense available for women: the choice to leave. Men know, Rosario professes, in a free union, that they must provide pleasure and care for women if they want the women to choose them, to capitulate. Rosario turns away from the narrator-protagonist, withdraws, and chooses another: "I kissed her, but she eluded me with a swift gesture, escaping from the arms that would embrace her, like an animal that does not want to be touched" (237). The jungle itself now closes up, submerging the signs of passage, denying access. Configured through a narrative of female resistance, interracial sexuality itself becomes the ultimate prohibition against reproduction.

But does it really?

The narrator-protagonist role as Latin American artist is intertwined with the line of his reproduction, his ability to assume the masculine through intercourse with the jungle, through bestowing a name on his creation of the "new." Critics, however, have remarked that the narrator-protagonist's sexual relations are repeatedly infertile, a conclusion that does not adequately explain the ambiguities in reproduction. Carmen Perilli, for example, insists that "in the story there are no biological children; instead they are only insinuated as a probability that gets frustrated" (94). And González Echevarría likewise claims:

> There are, in fact, no geneses in the novel, only repetitions, rediscoveries, and falsifications. When the protagonist begins to compose music in Santa Mónica, it is suggested that Rosario has become pregnant, but he never knows for sure, and then she marries Marcos. Ruth, his own wife, only feigns a pregnancy, and Mouche, his mistress, turns out to be a lesbian. Natural conceptions are fictional or nonexistent. (1977: 167)

However, the point missing from these interpretations is that the text allows the genesis while at the same time obstructing it. Upon his attempted return to the jungle, the narrator-protagonist learns from the Greek gold digger Yannes, when he inquires about Rosario, "Wife of Marcos ... she with child" (276). Yet, the date on the diary entry is 30 December, a Saturday, whereas the narrator-protagonist's departure from Santa Mónica appears to be sometime toward the middle of July, though the text does not register the exact date. Rosario's pregnancy signifies that he both succeeded in reproducing, in creating the "new," and did not. Symbolizing global integration in media networks and popular culture, interracial reproduction is posed, in *The Lost Steps,* as the absolute limit to difference and transformation and, at the same time, as their only possibility.

Carpentier's model of hybridity is not the only one available for thinking through different positions that the new cultures of globalization offer. Carpentier envisions the market and the media as fully flexible, able to integrate vast disparities and types into passionate friendships of communication. Such an understanding of the functioning of capital, unfortunately, is inadequate to account for the ways that markets and media are continually producing not only new enclaves of neglect and desperation but also new forces of resistance. In contrast, Angel Rama has traced Latin American history as a history of urbanity. As the center of power both political and religious, the Latin American city grew out of an inclination on the part of the colonizers and planners to order chaos through writing. The New World was to be the manifestation of a dream of utopian celestial order made real in concrete social spaces as proof of the rule of reason. Rama shows how this very meeting produced itself as a culture of critique. The collision between the European ideal and its representations on the one hand, and the reality of the Americas on the other, was established, according to Rama, as a site of hostile collisions, antagonisms, and contradictions remarked by the lettered classes themselves from inside of the power structure, as opposed to a site of loving synthesis and peaceful inclusion. In other words, the real itself was resistant to the ways that power and the media sought to represent it, enabling a powerful (if elite) public culture of radical democracy. The tradition of arts and philosophies in Latin America has therefore been always infused with a tendency toward oppositional critique. The implication is that one cannot assess the widespread extension of global communications as a culture of love, mutual benevolence, and feminine seductions but rather one of continual conflict.

What Rama's figuration contributes to the discussions of hybridity is the very real possibility of showing how migrant cultures are not just complicit in marrying themselves to, reproducing, and reinforcing the powers of capital but actually see themselves as necessarily in conflict with them. However, his project falls short in considering the practices of power. For one, his Habermasian view of the popular envisions an increasingly democratic culture of exchange—people meeting, for instance, in public spaces like coffeehouses—based in the autodidacticism of the urbanizing masses of the formally uneducated as well as the increasingly widespread access to print. "The confused and tumultuous process of democratization," explains Rama, "was creating a new type of letrado who, lacking contact with the most esteemed instrument of formal education, necessarily developed a less disciplined and systematic, but also more liberated, intellectual vision" (119). Intellectual and ideological thought accordingly became increasingly shaped by the demands of the lower classes, who were approaching the centers of power. This type of analysis projects culture onto a free-floating, abstracted, frictionless demand-and-supply curve, where the less powerful can assert claims and demand voice, representation, and remendation on the sheer force of their numbers. Historically, however, this has not proved the case. Surely not the audience dictates the content of ideology nor the modes of its operations but rather an elite few who control the venues of capital and communications.

The second shortcoming of Rama's history is this: it is clearly not the letter that imposes regulations and enforces draconian economic depravity on a population. He fails to mention that the letter is instituted presently through techniques of social control, including militarization, surveillance of and intelligence gathering on civilians, massacres, the terrorizing of the left, the imprisonment of political prisoners and oppositional groups, crop eradication, wars on drugs, federal austerity measures, governmental corruption, and so on—all forces of destruction and annihilation in league with global capitalism and neoliberal policies, as well as producers of violence and hunger. The construction of public space and democratic access in Latin America is not just the result of an intellectual exercise, designed in schools, libraries, and coffee shops, imagining social hierarchies of organization that will then materialize, but instead of a forceful reclaiming of the critical language of justice.

Mario Vargas Llosa and the Rape of Sebastiana

His desire had returned with a sort of mad fury and the baron bent down toward Sebastiana's vulva once again, pressing his face between her legs so as to separate them, forcing her to stretch out, so as to be able to kiss it again, breathe it in, sip it. He remained in that position for a long time, his eyes closed, intoxicated, taking his pleasure, and when he felt that he could no longer contain his excitement he straightened up, got onto the bed, and crawled on top of Sebastiana. Separating her legs with his, fumbling about for her privates with an uncertain hand, he managed to penetrate her in a moment that added pain and rending to his pleasure. He heard her moan, and managed to see, in the tumultuous instant in which life seemed to explode between his legs, that the baroness was still holding Sebastiana's face between her two hands, gazing at her with pity and tenderness as she blew gently on her forehead to free a few little hairs stuck to her skin.

—*The War of the End of the World*

... the one who supplants god is not only a symbolic assassin of reality, but, moreover, its thief. To suppress "her," "he" has to sack "her"; having decided to end with "her," "he" doesn't have any other remedy except always using "her." Thus, with respect to the material of "his" fictitious world, "he" is not even a creator; "he" appropriates, usurps, plunders immense reality, "he" converts "her" into his booty.[1]

—García Márquez, *Historia de un deicidio*

In 1990, novelist, essayist, and dermatologist Mario Vargas Llosa ran for president of Peru. For the coalition of party interests that he formed to support his candidacy and his program for economic and political reform, he coined the name "Libertad." Starting as a broad-based reaction against then-president Alan García's proposals to nationalize the Peruvian banking system in 1987, Libertad fashioned an agenda of economic neoliberalization. This involved the curtailment of state intervention in the market, ending the *assistentialismo* (nepotism) on all levels of the state bureaucracy, and the *modernización* of the domestic economy through its realignment within a transnational economic culture: basically, that is, through renegotiating the national debt, increasing exports, stabilizing exchange rates, privatizing national industries, offering credit guarantees to the agricultural sectors, instituting austerity programs and economic "shock" treatment (eliminating price ceilings), and lifting tariffs on trade—basically, the IMF platform.

Vargas Llosa's development of his aesthetic model of *libertad* in his 1981 novel *The War of the End of the World* foreshadows his presidential campaign's political platform of neoliberalization. Vargas Llosa's aesthetic "libertad" is loosely based on Bataille's theory of eroticism, a sacrifice within the economic order. The tale Vargas Llosa is telling about a group of marginal beggars and decrepit bandits, of Sebastianistas, who in 1898 rebel against the newly established Brazilian federation, disrupts the establishment of domesticity as the foundation of a new economic federalism. In one of the closing scenes of the novel, the Baron, assisted by his mad wife—both representatives of provincial power against centralization—rapes her mulatto servant Sebastiana. This triangulated, violent, primal scene of miscegenated penetration culminates the constant evocations, throughout the novel, of an illicit "intimacy" framing the relationship between the Baroness and Sebastiana. The plot of the Baroness and Sebastiana, shadowed with intimations of secrets going on in the recesses of domestic space, weaves a narrative of economic vitalization into a story about domestic relations. The Baroness's sterility, her absolute unreproductiveness *(libertad)* that is linked to failures in economic stability and market integration due to irrational and archaic institutions: feudal patronage, regional and familial allegiances, and the like. That the Baroness is cured of madness when her husband's position is restored through rape suggests that the health of the nation and the final leveling of the rebels who have resisted the law depend on the ultimate reconstitution of the domestic organization of gender in defense of civilization. The rebellion, a quest for full political autonomy and sovereignty, as it slides into a subtextually sexual narrative of relations between the landowning class and its domestic servants, generates itself as a sacred lawlessness, an absolute destructiveness to reproduction on the edge of a transition to a market economy. I here reconsider the political implications of using *la mestiza* as a figure for ethnic minority resistance and counterhegemonic literatures by showing how the same figure is rooted in Mario Vargas Llosa's global vision of economic reform. I look at the scene in *The War of the End of the World* where the Baron rapes Sebastiana as articulating a rebirth of nationalism and of a nationalist literature as a symbolic crux for new international relations of capital.

Beginning in the late 1960s, Vargas Llosa developed what might be called a theory of the novel based on a notion of *libertad* derived from Sartre's existentialism, Bataille's eroticism, and a loose interpretation of the romantic cult of the genius.[2] The artist as creator, as "supplanter of god" or "god-killer," according to Vargas Llosa, is in the business of destroying in order to recreate in his own subjective image "la realidad," or "ella": "To write novels," Vargas Llosa begins his critique of García Márquez (1971), "is an act of rebellion against reality, against God, against God's creation which is reality. It's a tentative correction, change or abolition of the real reality, and its substitution by a fictitious reality that the novelist creates" (85). The artist becomes, in this sense, self-generative and therefore free, outside the law. As Oviedo acknowledges, "Biological sterility, is, paradoxically, the guarantee for creative fecundity" (298). The rebellion against reality subjects the artist to seclusion, a separation between himself and others: "one declares oneself a *marginal* being" (95). The marginality and withdrawal of the artist is a consequence of reality's resistance to form, resulting in that the artist "feels deceived, betrayed, contradicted by reality" (92). In the act of creation, the artist "plunders" material from "la realidad real" (the real reality) in order to subject it to form.[3] In this way, the artist generates himself: "Having to 'invent himself,' left to his own forces, a quarry from which to extract literary and ideological materials useful for his vocation, is a difficult and painful enterprise, in which, at each step, he risks losing himself" (207). Becoming "a symbolic assassin of reality" (85), reaching into her to exploit what he finds, separating himself from her, rejecting her, smashing her, and rebelling against her, the artist painfully gives birth to himself.

The artist's self-birth is governed by an irrational subconscious impulse. Some event in the novelist's past lodges itself in his memory and destroys him. It is the nostalgia for this moment and the constant return to it that Vargas Llosa terms "el demonio," the demon. The novelist's only choice is to exorcise it, expel it, excrete it by giving it form. "El demonio" is where Vargas Llosa (1972) elides Bataille's theory of excess:

> The paradox of human life resides in that, to make possible the duration of being, to make life not cease, society has to constrain man, fence him in behind a wire mesh of taboos, obligate him to suffocate the non-rational part of his personality, that spontaneous and negative zone of his being which, if left in liberty, would destroy order. Eroticism . . . , sexual practice emancipated from reproduction, task essentially sterile, gratis, luxurious, wasteful, is one of those movements that are "tumultuous," "excessive," that oppose reason, the Good, and laboral activity, that is to say one of those privileged dominions of "*Evil and the diabolic*," thanks to which man, approaching death, can exercise his liberty, rebel and reach plenitude. ("Bataille O El rescate del Mal," 17–18)

"La libertad" is destructive of reality in order to affirm an autonomous space for the male desire for self-creation. It is an absolute unreproductiveness that opens the possibility of creation. It is the limit to reproduction that allows for its continuation. At the same time, therefore, for Vargas Llosa, the eroticism of "la libertad," the zone of destruction, is formulated as a baseline necessity for new production and innovation sustaining a national economy.

The absolute unreproductiveness so necessary, according to Vargas Llosa, for capitalist growth, produces the feminine as excess. For example, consumerism, advertising, and public relations, Vargas Llosa recognizes in *La orgía perpetua (The Perpetual Orgy),* his 1975 study on Flaubert, are fabricated as a story of a feminine desire for erotic lawlessness: "This abyss between desire and reality perhaps explains Emma's vocation to possess, her appetite for objects. . . . The case of Emma Bovary is a presage of that extraordinary phenomenon of the modern world whereby things, once the servants and instruments of mankind, become its masters and destroyers" (139–40). The idea that excessive consumption signifies, through the feminine, an excess of desire within the order of labor is already, in Bataille, a tenet of the destructive violence that, for him, is constitutive of capitalist accumulation: "That sparkling finery and that make-up," he writes in the second volume of *The Accursed Share,* "those jewels and those perfumes, those faces and those bodies dripping with wealth, becoming the *objects,* the focal points of luxury and lust, though they present themselves as goods and as values, dissipate a part of human labor in *useless* expenditure" (141). Absolute expenditure, outside of reproduction, outside the mechanization of labor, is what transforms the generative processes of literary creation, for Vargas Llosa, into a sacred sacrifice of "la realidad," a reproductive sterility linked to feminine desire.

In conformity with Vargas Llosa's own aesthetic declarations, much of the criticism on his literary work tends to focus on formal technique. Eduardo Béjar, for example, writes, "These texts carry deserved recognition for their formal innovations, and, as such, notable examples of a Latin American literature which claimed universal status" (243). The fragmentation of character, plot and setting, the layering of dialogues, the insertion of texts from popular culture, the attempts to create an epic totality in narrative form, the interweaving of multiple time frames, the use of autobiographical material, the precision of description and detail, the self-referential and nonself-referential intertextuality, the objectivity, the interaction of fiction and reality, and the proliferation of regional dialects, among other devices, direct critical attention toward a type of commentary concerned primarily with how Vargas Llosa's literary craft, as an experiment in realism, reflects Peruvian social reality through an obsession with form. In keeping with this, Oviedo remarks that "all the techniques concur with the realization of Vargas Llosa's well-established novelistic ideal: the dynamization of narrative reality to make it similar to the reality which is objective and captive to itself" (262). Much of the criticism, including Oviedo's own, attempts to unravel the complexity of the narrative structure in the various novels, separating out strains in the story, diagramming the patterns of chapters, deducing a chronology of events, and demonstrating how the structure of the narrative itself complicates the storytelling. However, his formal quality, so much flaunted by the critics and by Vargas Llosa himself, has lapses where it becomes evident that the propensity to systemic order, rigor, and control is so excessive because it rides on materials that resist this imposition.

Many critics have also observed that the resistance of the text to totalization arises from a demonic or unconscious (in the Freudian sense) emotional trauma. This trauma confronts, eludes, and suspends the rationality of technical and narrative control. Julio Ortega, for example, describes Vargas Llosa's novels as acts of seduction in that the novelist attracts and guides the reader "with the passion of his rigor which organizes itself like a strategy" (21). Nevertheless, Ortega goes on, "It is not casual that a form which is intensely systematic corresponds to a world of materials which are not systematic at all" (21–22). The critics who note this resistance, which interrupts the narrative and against which the narrative gets formed, usually follow Vargas Llosa's self-commentary by attributing them to "el Mal," the eroticism that Bataille alludes to in the interstices of social regulation.

What has not been particularly stressed, however, is that in Vargas Llosa's work this eroticism is often if not always tinged (and the argument could be made that Bataille's theory lends itself to this) with race and gender. In other words, eroticism arises or gets expressed when racial and gender categories suspend their rational organization. The two examples that Ortega gives of the perverse "questioning of models and codes" (23) are *La casa verde* (*The Green House,* 1966), where la Selvática, the indigenous girl kidnapped by nuns, becomes a prostitute, and *Conversación en la catedral* (*Conversation in the Cathedral,* 1969), where the collapse of organized political culture is elided into the brutal mutilation and murder of the lesbian prostitute. The rational imposition of narrative and technique is sustained through a regulation of gender and race.

In particular, *The War of the End of the World* is cited by critics as a novel whose narrative form is much more linear and tight, and whose technical experimentation is more minimal, than in his other works. For Keith Booker, "Vargas Llosa's treatment of this event [the rebellion in Brazil] lacks any obvious irony, parody, or reflexivity, and in fact seems to aspire to a straightforward retelling of the events in such a way that the writer's technique will be transparent and not interfere with the story being told" (75).

Raymond Leslie Williams agrees that "the novel seems traditional and even relatively simple. It is Vargas Llosa's only novel narrated extensively and consistently" (139). Timothy Brennan follows Benedict Anderson and Eric Hobsbawm in demonstrating how the absolute will to totality in narrative, in *The War of the End of the World,* is an attempt to invent a national community as a function of literary form, of print culture moving into a technological age.[4] Jean Franco, however, in "Self-Destructing Heroines," presents *The War of the End of the World* as an example of the "great historical novels of contemporary Latin America" (105) that separate women into conventional spaces: "Women in reality as well as in literature are overwhelmingly identified with fixed territories" (106).[5] Nevertheless, when Franco talks about the novel as separating the private from the public by regulating gender, she gives as an example—for women who, in crossing the boundaries, are debased by their exposure to the street—a passage from Arguedas that witnesses the street turned into a brothel by the presence of "blacks, mulattoes" (105). If the maintenance of narrative control relies on a strict segregation of racial and gender spheres of conduct, then eroticism, as it breaks down the border between rationality and primitivism, obstructs the closure of the narrative in conjugal resolution.

The saliency of Bataille's theory of eroticism for Vargas Llosa is in the way it plots the border between civilization and barbarism onto a sexually charged Hegelian engagement. Bataille's theory works under the supposition that capitalism is principled upon the impetus to accumulate excess and then dispense with it, rather than, upon a Malthusian model of limited resources and the competition over access to them, as in classical evolutionism. Erotism is life beyond utility, beyond necessity, an "abundance of resources" (1993, 162). Mixing Marxian dialectics with Durkheim and Mauss's sociology of the sacred, Bataille formulates this thesis within a developmental schema that starts with Aztec sacrifice, moves into potlatch rituals among the Kwakiutl and other Plains Indians, and shows how such sacred practices of destroying excess accumulation are worked inside, say, Cold War logic and the cultures of twentieth-century consumerism. As work and the rationality of labor draw the line between the primitive and the regime of rationality,[6] eroticism opens up rationalism to the regime of the primitive already inside: leisure, useless expenditure, sacrifice, and destruction. Eroticism, or excess, represents the chaotic, overwhelming, violent moment of dialectic synthesis, where subject and object, through death, reproduction, and/or the "urge to possess" (1986, 20), reach continuity or, as Bataille says, "the blending and fusion of separate objects" (25) showing "the significance of a barrier at the moment of its being overturned" (49).

The primitive sacred violence at the heart of Bataille's general economy—eroticism—is posed as the exterior limit to the rationality of the subject under capitalism. Female sexuality becomes the prism through which primitive excess and sacred violence are imagined as the object of rational control. Thus, femininity, in Bataille's theory, is constantly being evoked as a racial category. The subjective fusion is woven into a story of feminine violation:

> The passive, female side is essentially the one that is dissolved as a separate entity. But for the male partner the dissolution of the passive partner means one thing only: it is paving the way for a fusion where both are mingled, attaining at length the same degree of dissolution. The whole business of eroticism is to destroy the self-contained character of the participators as they are in their normal lives. (17)

The feminine represents the intrusions of savagery within the laboral order. Situated as the absolute unreproductiveness, as the violence and destruction that establishes dialectical synthesis and capitalist modes of accumulation through primitive excess, the feminine is created through racial discourse, as it is in Vargas Llosa's work.

In *The War of the End of the World*, Vargas Llosa employs the body of the mixed-blood woman, Sebastiana the *macuma*, as both the telling symbol of national (and sexual) unity and narrative adhesion, and as a rebellion against civic order, a deviant resistance signifying the disintegration of institutions (including civil marriage and literature). Much lesbian theory, following Gloria Anzaldúa's extraction from the figure of the *mestiza* as expressing the possibility of liberation, has focused on the mixed-blood woman's resistance to categorization as a potential for exploring an emancipatory deconstruction of sexual identities and subjectivities in the limits of racial representation. Anzaldúa has reworked, critics such as Judith Raiskin contend, the fixed categories of racial, sexual, and national identity from nineteenth-century evolutionary science, particularly of "the essentialist language of Krafft-Ebing's "psychic hermaphrodite" and Carpenter's "intermediate sex" (161). Anzaldúa's "own vision," argues Raiskin, "challenges the modernist longing for unity and cohesiveness" and "embodies a continual confrontation of differences, a 'crossbreeding' that allows 'for a preservation under a variety of conditions'" (163). Vargas Llosa's appropriation of a similar symbolic structure, though, necessitates a further look at the historical vectors that converge in the body of the *mestiza* and complicate the possibility of her symbolic mobilization within or as an emancipatory project.

Anzaldúa's focus on the *mestiza* as a cultural-symbolic challenge to structural mechanisms of oppression and to a hierarchical ordering of humanity furnishes, Anzaldúa proclaims, a method for transcending, through mixing, the reification of the language of identity:

> The U.S.-Mexican border *es una herida abierta* where the Third World grates against the first and bleeds. And before a scab forms it hemorrhages again, the lifeblood of two worlds merging to form a third country—a border culture. Borders are set up to define the places that are safe and unsafe, to distinguish *us* from *them.* A border is a dividing line, a narrow strip along a steep edge. A borderland is a vague and undetermined place created by the emotional residue of an unnatural boundary. It is in constant state of transition. The prohibited and forbidden are its inhabitants. *Los atravesados* live here: the squint-eyed, the perverse, the queer, the troublesome, the mongrel, the mulato, the half-breed, the half dead; in short, those who cross over, pass over, or go through the confines of the "normal." (3)

However, by constantly evoking blood metaphors, Anzaldúa's scheme tends to close in on itself, reinstituting the very biology that a so-called revolutionary approach to identity would seem to dislodge. As such, Anzaldúa's experiment falls back into essentialist paradigms: the *mestiza* would travel from one blood-based identity to another, crossing borders on either side of which the definitional configurations remain intact, inhabiting one at a time, always guided through one or another strain of her bloodline. What AnnLouise Keating notes as "revisionist mythmaking," an "agent of transformation" serving "to displace the conventionalist boundaries between inner/outer, subject/object, and self/other" (87), can just as easily function as a reinstatement of these same boundaries where the creator can jump over the dividing line into the alternative setting, without ever causing any kind of serious wounding or transformation in the systemic locations and categories of bodies. Anzaldúa, for instance, performs such acrobatics with her dualistic linguistic registers. The use of Spanish phrases thrown into the middle of English sentences or interrupting the linguistic unity of a prosaic or poetic line, splitting it between the two different sign systems of the divided *mestiza* identity, is heavily weighted toward an Anglo-identified readership: the Spanish is rendered in italics and is often translated in footnotes or immediately subsequent to the phrase. (The English is never translated.) The Spanish speech is therefore the outside, the object, and the other—the "real"—as the blood flows back to a nostalgic geography of lexical simplicity within a hierarchical organization. Not only that, but the linguistic mixing seems to offer a purely culturalist understanding of border mixing. There is no sense of how power and money, rather than desire or a free-floating language, control passage through the border.

The shoebox mapping of identities in space, which the figure of the border solidifies *and* transforms, leads to an idealization of the racial roots of conquest and, in particular, to a reduction of the Indian past into a primitive or originary freedom—a rebellion. "My Chicana identity," she says, "is grounded in the Indian woman's history of resistance" (21). This confiscation of Indianness for a revolutionary spiritualism of queerness slots the figure of the Indian in a preconquest landscape, overly simplistic, ahistorical, atemporal, and rhetorical:

> I've always been aware that there is a greater power than the conscious I. That power is my inner self, the entity that is the sum total of all my reincarnations, the godwoman in me I call *Antigua, mi Diosa*, the divine within, *Coatlicue-Cihuacoatl-Tlazolteotl-Tonantzin-Coatlalopeuh-Guadalupe.* (50)

The Indian becomes a mystical leitmotif invoked as a discursive tool, an objectified incarnation of the deconstructive indeterminacy and the utopic politics that the border is supposed to promise. And it is through this claiming of an Indian soul that the *mestiza* artist can create: "The ability of story (prose and poetry) to transform the storyteller and the listener into something or someone else is shamanistic. The writer, as shape-changer, is a *nahual*, a shaman" (1987: 66). In an act of rebellion, the *mestiza* claims Indianness as a source of female sexuality: "The Third World Woman revolts: *We revoke, we erase your white male imprint. When you come knocking on our doors with your rubber stamps to brand our faces with DUMB, HYSTERICAL, PASSIVE PUTA, PERVERT, when you come with your branding irons to burn MY PROPERTY on our buttocks, we will vomit the guilt, self-denial and race-hatred you have force-fed into us right back into your mouth*" (1981: 167). Miscegenation frames the birth of a nation of Third World women writers, of nation as literature.

In fact, the construction of "America" and of "American national literature" around the concept of difference and a plurality of possible racial identifications has traditionally formed the groundwork for symbolizing national culture in the same U.S. and Hispanic patriarchal cultures from which Anzaldúa tries to separate and differentiate her "new" *mestiza* identity. As George Yúdice has pointed out, multiculturalism's ambitions in "claiming to represent the numerous perspectives of peoples around the world" echoes a pretension particularly emblematic of U.S. histories of self-definition, the nation's self-fashioning as a "microcosm of the world" (202), as a "land of immigrants" or "melting pot"; as Ella Shohat has demonstrated, "multiplicity," "syncretism," and "hybrid cultures" "had already been invoked decades ago by diverse Latin American modernisms" (108). But Klor de Alva vituperates what he calls "Latin American mainstream's narrative on *mestisaje*" (1992: 5) for its overwhelming turn toward Europeanized cultural practices at the expense of indigenous recognition. Similarly, Román de la Campa has questioned the tendency, on the part of literary criticism and Hispanic writings of *mestizaje*, to place Hispanic writings at the center of the West's search for an epistemic absence in order to "prove" postmodernity's decentering of the subject and referential uncertainties: "Errancy, absence, lack of a center, confusion, search for identity, desire to name the abyss—all become signifiers that govern and inform Latin American literature and writing" (1995: 760). Anzaldúa's revisioning of *mestiza* as identity (both ethnic/national and literary), such criticism would insinuate, is repeating a critical tendency to use Latin America and particularly Latin American women as a pure referential sign while idealizing its nationalist symbols as the "reality" of liberatory valor on the margins of postmodernity.

Thus, *mestiza* consciousness, even as it might allow for temporal displacements of a univocal conception of self, does not only profess harmony in multiplicity. Nor does it necessarily, as Yvonne Yarbro-Bejarano contends, "challenge . . . the dominant male concepts of cultural ownership and literary authority" (733). Criticizing lesbian critics such as Yarbro-Bejarano, who uphold the border as site of a radical politics of hybridization, Annamarie Jagose rereads Anzaldúa and finds the border undermining the project of confluence and harmonious integration that the same border would seem to construct:

> This valorization of the border as the site of linguistic or generic confluence, which necessarily represses the opposite facet of the border as a site of linguistic or generic demarkation, is itself structured by that repression. For, in the terms of *Borderlands'* own argument, intermixture is possible only where there is segregation. The attempt to celebrate the Chicano's location as a linguistic and genetic switchpoint, a point of evolutionary conflux, is undermined by the insistent return of repressed notions of partition and division which equally characterize his position:
>
> *¿Quién está tratando de cerrar la fisura entre la india y el blanco en nuestra sangre? El Chicano, sí, el Chicano que anda como un ladrón en su propia casa* (63). (155)

The *mestiza* is a social production generated by a series of segregated histories that converge and come apart again, divided into racial and gender dichotomies as much as the *mestiza* also conflates these divisions. The figurative body of the *mestiza*, in its multiple deployments and shifting categories of cultural practice, can function as an embodiment of a genealogy of conquest, marginalization and genocide, a doubled signifier encoding a conflict in its multiple historical dimensions. The utopic tendency, evinced in recent lesbian theory such as Raiskin's, Yarbro-Bejarano's, and Keating's, to idealize her into a formulaic buzzword for a subversive deregulation and destabilization of races, sexualities, literatures, and nationalities neglects the fact that such an idealization repeats the painful legacy of forced labor and forced migration of peoples who might claim residence on the other side of that border. The border, then, masks by assimilating the real politics of colonialism as well as the current power structure that uses Indians for, say, underpaid manufacturing labor or cash-based domestic service without contracts or benefits. It constructs an objectified, ethereal, gendered, and atemporal image of a partitioned-off Indianness that can again be subjected to somebody else's political agenda. Envisioning a world made up of disappearing borders, *mestiza* consciousness, like the ideologies of global capitalism, thinks freedom as a product of deregulation, allowing capital to access other nations without allowing free passage for everybody.

Because *mestizaje* creates hierarchical separation and, at the same time, a site of fusion, it can operate as an insignia of redemption while still exalting a justificatory story for racist and sexist oppressions. The flip-side, the figure of the mixed-blood woman as a cultural and literary product of oppressive nationalisms and imperial relations, has been overlooked among lesbian theorists who are rushing toward her to claim her as a symbolic structure for a new radicalism. In Latin American letters, the mixed-blood woman is the one contaminated by the blood of conquest. She originates *la raza*, the *mestizo* community that constitutes the nation, in rape. Tracing the history of Mexican usage of the verb *chingar*, Octavio Paz explains that "the verb denotes violence, an emergence from oneself to penetrate another by force. It also means to injure, to lacerate, to violate—bodies, souls, objects—and to destroy" (76–77). Carlos Fuentes works Paz's *chingada* into a symbol for the unity of bourgeois ideology and capitalist cohesion, within which Mexico's multiple races are contained. Fuentes is talking here about the postrevolutionary moment in Mexico, where the *mestizo* middle classes assumed mediating positions in an international politics of investment and a revitalization of economic and State liberalization:

> Born of fucking, dead from fucking, living fucked: pregnant belly and winding sheet, hidden in the word. It faces you everywhere, it deals your hand, cuts your deck, covers your bet, disguises reticence and the double-cross, reveals cowardice and bravery, intoxicates, shouts, succumbs, lives in every bed, presides over the ceremonies of friendship, of hatred and of power: our word, you and I, members of the lodge, the fraternity of the fucked: you are what you are because you knew how to fuck 'em without letting them fuck you; you are what you are because you didn't fuck around: chain-gang of the fucked, linked before and behind, joined to all who have lost and preceded us, to all who will lose and follow. (138)

The *mestizo* is born out of a woman who is perverse in her prostitution, a traitor to her race (la Malinche often undergirds the referent), and yet reappropriated as an originary coordinate whose racial source is erased in the celebration of economic integration. The blood metaphor, while allowing for a plurality of positions, creates a collapse, becomes a symbol of national fusion inasmuch as the various bloodlines merge into a unity that obliterates the divergence of alternative blood histories. The mixed-blood woman, therefore, as Anzaldúa says of the lesbian, has paradoxically no race (80) because she is of all races. Vargas Llosa's character Sebastiana carries with her a literary tradition foregrounding sexual violation, where this violation is idealized as the founding moment of a liberal nation of *mestizos*, a moment of inclusion through forgetting, of deracialization in a utopian cultural unification, a salvation through economic internationalism. "Peruvian reality is, then," comments Nélida Flórez, "the continuation of the *original encounter* and the forgetting of the Inca or Spanish past. Vargas Llosa is a product of this mixing" (42).

The mixed-blood woman, then, presages a rift in the romance of domestic integrity, which Doris Sommer says constitutes the symbolic origin of a Latin American nationalist imaginary: "Erotic passion was [in post-Independence nineteenth century Latin American writings] less the socially corrosive excess that was subject to discipline in some model novels from Europe, and more the opportunity (rhetorical and otherwise) to bind together heterodox constituencies: competing regions, economic interests, races, religions" (14). Domestic organization became the tension toward which narrative plots would build, Sommer observes, because "romantic novels go hand in hand with patriotic history in Latin America. The books fueled a desire for domestic prosperity; and nation-building projects invested private passions with public purpose.... Romance and republic were often connected" (7). However, the twentieth century witnessed a cynicism in the postindependence assimilationist ideal of sentimentalist national adhesion. As Sommer argues, the closure of nineteenth-century plots in marriage came to represent a nation-building that was symbolic, closed off from the influences of foreign philosophies and immigration (51) and constituted by "associative behavior, unfettered market relationships, and ... Nature in general" (35). Yet, in the twentieth century, it became clear that the market failed to equalize social relations, implement justice, or end violence. The disintegration of narrative homemaking and heterosexual union, as the nationalist project is perpetually postponed, comes to reside, as Vargas Llosa's Sebastiana demonstrates, in the image of the mixed-blood woman who, as a guest in the house, blocks the closure of the nationalist narrative by reinsinuating the repressed histories of rape, conquest, economic exploitation, social fragmentation, cultural exclusion, and bureaucratic breakdown into the foundational contract.

In late nineteenth-century Peruvian discourses on women, discussion of the domestic was concerned with guarding racial purity. The home, with the wife/mother as its guiding force, was supposed to uphold civilization.[7] Part of the debate focused on whether women should be educated and, if so, in what way. Women's education, masculinist polemicizers claimed, would cause the destruction of the political base of the country and a moral collapse. The intellectual work of women was seen to threaten civilization at its foundations by undermining morality; if women were educated, they would be more likely to enter public life at the expense of the home. In response, women argued that civilization would only be secured if women were educated because they would be less likely to stray from the home and that women's writing would constitute the culmination of her maternal-conjugal role in the passing on of civilized values. In 1874, for example, Mercedes Cabello de Carbonera wrote:

> The instruction and morality of women has been in every epoch the thermometer which has marked the progress and the degree of civilization and virility of nations. . . . Educate the woman, demonstrate her intelligence, and you will have in her a powerful and universal motor for the progress and civilization of the world, and a strong and irremovable column in which to cement the moral and virtues of the generations to come. (89–90)

The terms in which such women defended themselves did not put into question the role of domestic duty in maintaining civilization but instead repositioned learning as a way for the middle-class domestic wife/mother to strengthen the home, through abolishing the decadence of leisure, against racial backsliding. For example, in the same article, Cabello stated, "The reform which we would like to see realized in the education of the woman, does not distance her from the domestic home, but instead, on the contrary, gives it one more attraction, surrounding her with the enchantment of knowledge, which makes laziness inaccessible, this sickness, this nostalgia of the soul, which sterilizes life" (145–46). As Martiza Villavicencio sums up the controversy over women's education, "The treatment which is given to the woman is one of the signs by which one can tell the difference between a civilized society and a barbaric one" (39).

In actuality, Vargas Llosa is participating in this streamlining of femininity as a border marking the difference between civilization and barbarism. Within this positioning of the domestic wife/mother as the marker of civilization's stability lies a colonial legacy that casts indigenous and mulatto women as contrary and even menacing to romances of domestic closure. During the colonial era, discussions of concubinage, at least in part, participated in constructing race around discourses of colonial authority. According to the Peruvian historian Pablo Macera, the Indian uprisings of the eighteenth century, along with economic deflation, made it apparent to *criollo* nobles that contrary to the "prejuicios de sangre," it would be impossible to maintain families (326). The turn toward other forms of sexual conduct was an economic necessity, but the practice clearly corresponded with the conception that the popular classes were, as a condition, less disciplined, weaker in paternal authority, and therefore more promiscuous (339). Macera goes on to explain how, because of their link to disease and contamination, extramarital arrangements came to represent "causes and symptoms simultaneously of a decomposition which debilitated all of Peruvian society of the eighteenth century" (343). Marriage was thus defined against the popular classes, composed of Indian and mulatto moralities, to keep the order and guard the stability of the national social fabric, protecting the civilized home from barbarous influences.

The idea that black, Indian, or mulatto women threatened domestic controls on white women's bodies may be traced to the period when Peru was moving from colonialism to independence. Analyzing representations of the *tapadas* ("upper class women who covered their heads and face as a means of escaping surveillance by their families and husbands" [333]) at the beginning of the period of independence, Deborah Poole notes how the disguise itself created an aura of seduction around women in the veil. Their very entrance into the public arena granted them a visibility that, in women, could only circulate as sensuality and licentiousness. In order to signify this desire in women whose sexuality was supposed to be submerged in family structures and hidden in reproductive life, illustrators often placed them in marketplace settings where the figures could interact with popular types. Poole writes,

> This image of *tapadas* as conversing or otherwise engaging in social commerce with women of the lower orders, was very much part of their mystique. It was through such transactions that the *tapada* situated herself squarely in the midst of a public life seen by Europeans to be perilously close to the exposed and highly maternal womanhood of the *mulatta*, as symbol of disorder and sexual disease. . . . Largely through their association with the open market and the principle of barter (seen as a means of forcing social or conversational interaction between buyer and seller), maternity and female physiology became associated . . . with images of filth, depravity, and the aggressive nature of lower class sexuality. (348–49)

The appearance of the *tapadas* coincided with a particularly troublesome time in Peruvian history, when Peru was first defining itself as a nation. The ruling *criollo* elite, having recently beaten Spain in its struggle for independence, sought to maintain legitimacy by reinstituting the class and racial hierarchies of the colonial period. According to Poole, this process was significantly allied with the regulation of gender:

> Peruvian *criollo* men were, for the most part, confidently embarked on the formation of a new republic, in which they would play the role of mercantile brokers. . . . Upper-class coastal women, by comparison, had a much more intimate relationship with the Indian and black servants with whom they lived, and on whose services the *criollo* class depended. . . . Following a war in which "Peruvians" had been called up to liberate themselves as a group from Spain, continuing "intimacy" with their black and Indian compatriots was increasingly perceived as threatening to a class whose continuing economic dominance depended on constructing and maintaining the racial hierarchies of *colonial* Peru. (361)

Representing the border between races that holds colonial power in place, the privacy and unknowability of the *tapada*—a primary image of the domestic organization at the heart of republican nationhood—is transacted through the public visibility of a multiracial market life with which she is "intimate."

The historical situation of the mixed-blood woman in Peru, and all the associations she embodies, reflect the difficulties of assimilating her into a liberating politics for transcending identity. Essentially, in this context (which, I would emphasize, is different than Anzaldúa's), she is the white woman's ghost, her excess, the one whose contiguous existence endangers the white woman's reproduction of the line between civilization and barbarism. Sebastiana marks the boundary where gender identities are socially drawn through heterosexual binaries, as well as the possibility of opening the domestic into public circulation. The subversion that her multiple locations might generate becomes instead, as Judith Butler offers, a complex site for both "constraining and constituting the very possibilities of volition" (1990: 124).

The War of the End of the World is centered in the citadel of Canudos, where the rebels have congregated to defend the religious and antirepublican teachings of Antonio Consejero against the incursions of first the Bahían military and then the Brazilian armed forces. In support of the Portuguese imperial king, whom he sees as the soldier of Christ and his church and the abolisher of slavery,[8] el Consejero tears up the tax ordinances sent from the capital and, in this gesture, inaugurates a Catholic community that would also refuse the centralized governmental authority's imposition of statistical maps, the census, the metric system, and civil marriage. All these things, he preaches, are maneuvers of the antichrist, the Protestant republic announcing the apocalypse. For the advocates inside, the purpose of Canudos was to create an isolated community of resistant believers ruled by the paternalistic authority of el Consejero, personally allied, defensively enclosed, self-sufficient, and untouched by national infiltration.

The story germinates in a set of concentric circles that turn around this center. The ramifications of the conflict in Canudos are explored through the exposition of different points of view of the different people who are affected, internally or externally, by the uprising. The further away from this center the character is positioned, the more unintelligible the events at Canudos appear, and the more difficult it is for the character to decipher the message of Canudos. In fact, the forth and final book of the novel is composed of a set of flashbacks interspliced within a dialogue taking place between the Baron and the myopic journalist who had taken refuge inside the citadel and who was planning to write a book about it but, having broken his glasses, had not been able to see what had been happening around him.[9] The exchange circulates around the question of Canudos as the two interlocutors try to interpret the history that keeps eluding them: Was it a monarchical plot? A plot of the British, whose economic interests in Brazil were protected by the Portuguese crown? A plot of Epaminondas Gonçalves, leader of the opposition Partido Republicano Pregresista, to undermine the Baron's regional power and factionalize his Autonomist Party? An international conspiracy? Simply an irrational cry of desperation among the downtrodden, or an explosion of passion among religious fanatics? Was it organized and commissioned by the church? Or by a sector of the church?[10] Where this conversation terminates without resolution, the Baron, suddenly afflicted with passion and desire, climbs the stairs to his wife's bedroom and rapes Sebastiana.

Two of the few main characters who are radically affected by the rebellion at Canudos but whose interior consciousnesses are not entered into and dissected by the narrative are, significantly, the Baroness and Sebastiana. The Baron's desire for an end to the indeterminable narrative of Canudos slides into his sexual desire for Sebastiana, who has become an unintelligible exclusion within the novel's own logic. In this regard, the question that Galileo Gall, the Scottish phrenologist revolutionary, the ironical self-proclaimed "cambatiente de la libertad" (20), asks as he approaches Canudos (he dies before arriving), is particularly resonant: "Was he about to die," he thinks, "on account of such a stupid thing as a woman's cunt?" (292).[11] The way Canudos, throughout the novel, in many different of the trajectories, merges into an unconsummated sexual desire would pose the call to Canudos (and "libertad") as an epistemological problem set into a plot of female flight: the desire to reach Canudos, to see it and to know it and finally to die for it—the impossible desire, that is, to close it in narration, is interlocked with the male desire for the resistant woman, the one who destroys him by damaging his household and his honor.

Similar to what Béjar observes of *La historia de Mayta* (1984) and *La Ciudad y los perros* (1963), the irreducible language that is Canudos (and "libertad") is symbolized in the "lack," that is, "by means of the allegorization of the woman as discourse of resistance to the *will to truth* implicit in the power/control of the authorial intentionality and critical reading" (245). For Vargas Llosa, the hole that is woman, the wound to masculine honor that blocks his arrival, his mastery, and his knowledge and eventually destroys him—*libertad*—is further elided into a figure of femininity that, referencing racial exoticism, undermines the very claims to domesticity that she, at the same time, embodies. Waving her magic wand, Vargas Llosa writes in his essay "La cultura de la libertad," "la libertad" is revered and obeyed, despite her magic spells, her fanaticisms, her fetishistic whims, and inflicted sufferings (442). "Liberty, nutritive source of the best that has happened to man and his most costly yearning, is also an abyss down which he can roll and destroy himself" (437). Elided into the primitive violence of the sacred, *libertad* recreates domesticity as generative, nutritive, *and* destructive.

Woven as a series of strong narrative lines that are constantly intersecting, the plots of *The War of the End of the World* themselves are structured as enclosures continually infracted. Each character's subjectivity is a self-contained module of story that is, at the same time, merging with other settings and sites of consciousness. The many parallels between the many different offshoots of the central plot create a constant shifting between the inside and the outside of the core story at Canudos. The impossibility of telling Canudos rests on the difficulty of finding a position from which to tell it but also on the resistance of the material itself, that is, on the way the material is always betraying the one who wants to tell it by constantly shifting ground, becoming elusive, and breaking away from the formal grasp of each particular narrator. For instance, the Baron's uncontrollable desire, just before he rapes Sebastiana, is shadowed by an earlier scene: Galileo Gall rapes Jurema, wife of the tracker Rufino, after years of keeping an oath of abstinence for the sake of the revolution, initiating his pilgrimage to Canudos. The two scenes are so interconnected they resist closure, as Gall's story has elements that surface within the Baron's narrative: "The things he had been afraid of as he approached," he ruminates as he holds down Sebastiana,

> —what would the servant's reaction be? what would Estela's be if Sebastiana woke up screaming?—disappeared instantly and, as startling as a hallucination, the face of Galileo Gall flashed before his mind and he remembered the vow of chastity that the revolutionary had sworn to himself in order to concentrate his energies on things he believed to be of a higher order—action, science.... Without ever having sworn to do so, he had kept a similar vow for a very long time, renouncing pleasure. (536)

The crossing of the Baron's narrative with Galileo Gall's, though not the only instance of this kind of character merging in the novel,[12] exemplifies interconnections and splitting between different spatial and subjective divisions in the novel.

Interpenetrating and foreshadowing the ultimate destruction of the Baron's *hacienda* by the rebels of Canudos, Jurema's story is essentially an exploration of the quest for masculine honor shattered by a woman's betrayal, flight and resistance, her rape by Gall and the subsequent burning of her home. Conjointly, the loss of honor precipitates a turn toward Canudos and a continuously obstructed desire to get inside of it, to know it. After her rape, Jurema's flight incites the tracker and her husband Rufinos who, in his desire for vengeance, burns her house and chases her toward Canudos. Gall and Rufino die fighting each other en route; Jurema finally arrives but disappears from the text with no notice and no explanation.

Motivating the narrative movement is Jurema's position as a rupture in masculine honor and in the narrative cohesion, which significantly points back to her upbringing in Estela's household and in the triangle of resentment and jealousy that the three women lived out in the seclusion of the Baroness's bedroom:

> Once again the baron was overcome by the feeling that it was all unreal, a dream, a fiction, which always took possession of him at the very thought of Canudos. . . . The baron felt a desire to see Jurema again; perhaps it would do the baroness good to see this girl toward whom she had shown such affection in bygone days. He remembered that Sebastiana had felt a veiled resentment toward her for that very reason, and recalled how relieved she had been to see her go off to Queimadas with Rufino. (502)

Again the question arises, What was going on inside?—but this time in reference to the portrait of "intimacy" between the mistress and her servants in the privacy and isolation of a ruling-class home. The old patriarchal economic order that the Baroness represents here slides into, in the Baron's memory, the unfathomability, the irreducibility, the blindness that is Canudos.

The loss of masculine honor and the subsequent quest to reclaim it create a tension, a narrative tension riding on the desire to know, a tension signified through the inability (in the text's own terms) of either Jurema or the Baroness to bear children. Rufino tracks down Jurema at the ambush in Caracatá, where she played the role of a prostitute to lure the Seventh

Regiment soldiers so that the rebels, silently approaching, could corner them. Having at last found her and tied her up (later he will lead her around on a leash), Rufino explains why the rape and the quest, staining his honor, have obsessed and changed him: "You have a milk inside you now that isn't mine. I know now why God punished you for so long, not letting you get pregnant" (275). Jurema's barrenness, as a result of her insult to masculine honor—her possession by another man, her flight—crosses into the narrative of Estela's own sterility. Just as Rufino's home was burned when he learned of his wife's betrayal—her rape by Gall as representative of "libertad"—precipitating their flight to Canudos, Calumbí, their *hacienda,* has been burned by the rebels, and the Baron and Baroness have been forced to flee. As a result, the Baroness has gone insane: "'Those flames are still burning here inside me.' She touched her stomach and doubled over, trembling. 'It was as though the children I lost when they were born were being burned to cinders'" (277). For the Baroness, the original betrayal, one that precipitates her husband's loss of honor, is a betrayal of the domestic, which she has left in ruins, but also a betrayal within the domestic, her absolute unreproductivity. The difference between the stories of the servant class heading toward Canudos, and the land-holding ruling classes moving away, is fused into the symbolic production of endangered domesticity and of feminine betrayal in unreproductivity.

The first thing the Baron thinks about, when the bandit Pajeú, the "half-breed" messenger and representative of Canudos, announces that Calumbí will be burned, is Sebastiana: "He was suddenly moved by the desire to penetrate . . . to know the secret roots. . . . And at the same time there came to his mind's eye the image of Sebastiana brushing Estela's fair hair amid a circle of flames. The color drained from his face" (245). The desire to know Canudos leads to a desire to open, to know, the domestic closure as the space of reproduction. The presence of Sebastiana in the Baron's imagination at this moment merges what happens in the Baroness's bedroom with the unreproductivity of Canudos. The Baron cannot possibly understand or penetrate the violence that will destroy his home, the violence of Canudos, just as he cannot understand the "intimacy" between the Baroness and the servant class, the originating betrayal, the unreproductivity.

The dimness and confusion of knowledge that the violence of Canudos represents is thus evoked through allusions to the secret collusion of classes and races framing the Baroness's bedroom, sexuality, and reproductive body. The Baron's entrance into the Baroness's bedroom, where he would rape Sebastiana, is precipitated in shadows, light and darkness, which inhibit his complete mastery of access and comprehension. At first, the Baron is worried lest the very walls of the chambers block the attainment of his desire: "As his hand reached out toward the latch, the thought occurred to him that the door might be locked" (536). When the door gives way, the very space into which the Baron penetrates is fractured into partial illuminations that allow only Sebastiana's body to come into view as fragments and distortions of form. Standing above Sebastiana and looking down on her, "from the doorway he spied the yellow light of the night lamp—a candlewick floating in a little bowl of oil—whose dim light illuminated part of the baroness's bed. . . . He reached the edge of her [Sebastiana's] bed without awakening her. There was a dim light in the room—the glow from the gas lamp out in the street, which took on a blue tinge as it filtered through the curtains—and the Baron could make out the woman's sleeping form" (536).

The deformation of Sebastiana's body and identity parallels the reformation of the Baroness out of the deformity of sickness and irrationality. When she approaches Sebastiana's bed, lightly intrigued, the Baroness "was wearing a light nightdress, beneath which he could dimly make out in the half light the faint outlines of her body, which time had not contrived to deform" (539). Only the ends of her hair, which the text constantly describes as touched and combed by Sebastiana, are still shrouded outside the light. Reminiscent of the deformations of the reality of Canudos, which the myopic journalist, having lost his glasses, desires to form into narrative, this moment is when the Baron declares his love for his wife, reaffirming his marriage vows, and says that his rape of Sebastiana is for the good and the health of the Baroness.

In an uncanny presentiment of what would occur in his own home, the Baron, when Pajeú announces the destruction of Calumbí, foretells the violence Canudos was to spark in his domestic security: "It was as if the world had taken leave of its reason and blind, irrational beliefs had taken over" (246). Canudos is the externalization of the Baroness's mind and body, what her enclosure in the domestic occluded. As such, the capitulation of Canudos is steeped in the flames that consume the Baroness's womb, exposing Canudos as the absolute negation of reproductivity. In the scene between the one describing the rape and the one presenting the last battle cry, the ceasefire, of Canudos, the Léon de Natuba—the hunchbacked scribe of the now-dead Consejero—immolates himself, carbonizing himself in the flames of the last falling buildings and the last bombardment. The leveling of Canudos and the end of its narrative are envisioned through the complete deformation and fragmentation of the bodies inside the house in an act of sacrifice, each one fighting to death. Climbing the stairs on his way to rape Sebastiana, the Baron remembers what the Colonel Murau had told him about his last sighting of Canudos in ruins:

> They realized that the sound was that of the flapping wings and pecking beaks of thousands upon thousands of vultures, of that endless sea of grayish, blackish shapes covering everything, devouring everything, gorging themselves, finishing off, as they sated themselves, what neither dynamite nor bullets nor fires had been able to reduce to dust: those limbs, extremities, head, vertebras, viscera, skin that the conflagration had spared or only half charred and that these rapacious creatures were now crushing to bits, tearing apart, swallowing, gulping down. "Thousands upon thousands of vultures," Colonel Murau had said. (534–35)

The Baron's approach to Sebastiana, her visual dismemberment in the flickering flame of a candle and a streetlamp, is doubled in the vision of a completely demolished Canudos. The fires burning in Estela's womb, then, and at the end of Canudos, are doused in a narrative of masculine re-possession, powers of generation, and national honor.

Sebastiana's "intimacy" with the Baroness, as an absolute destruction of reproductivity, initiates the processes by which literature, the telling of Canudos, can be created. In 1967, receiving el Premio Internacional de Literatura Rómulo Gallegos in Caracas for his novel *La casa verde*, Vargas Llosa devised a position for the writer at the time Latin American nations were starting to recognize the value of their literatures in nation-building processes:

> To warn [Latin Americans] that literature is fire, that it signifies nonconformity and rebellion, that the *raison d'être* for the writer is protest, contradiction and criticism. Nobody who is satisfied is capable of writing, nobody who is in agreement, reconciled with reality, would commit the ambitious foolishness of inventing verbal realities. The literary vocation is

> born from the disagreement of a man with the world, from intuition, from deficiencies, from empty spaces and waste around him. (134–35)

Reality is figured in a constant rebellious flight, inciting the desire of the artist to create in pursuit of it, the desire for the irreconcilable object. National literature is a fire, even a volcanic explosion, which depends upon the artist's abstinence from intercourse with it and destroys absolutely the reproduction of it. In *La guerra del fin del mundo*, Vargas Llosa places this sacrificial fire within the ruling-class domestic enclosure, the space of femininity, while representing this absolute unreproductivity and complete unknowability within the history of the rebellion at Canudos: the way it resists comprehension and totalization in narrative and national cohesion, the way that women flee toward it—endlessly—as men pursue them through trajectories of desire, the way that fires that consume it at the end. The many sites of absolute unreproductivity—of the internal resistance inciting the formation of a national literature—in *La guerra del fin del mundo* fuse into three final images: one, a privatized and veiled "intimacy" between races of women; two, a sacrifice in fire; and three, a magisterial domination, through sex, of black female servant by a white landowner, a member of the governing elite.

The idea that racial mixture would become a metaphor for the production of a Peruvian national literature is not new to Vargas Llosa and, actually, has been firmly entrenched in the political ideologies of the Peruvian left. For example, Jose Carlos Mariátegui, who founded the Peruvian Communist Party (PCP) in 1923, stated that Peruvian literature would evolve into an indigenous realist literature that would be composed of a dualism, a mixture between Spanish (criollism) and indigenous (indigenist) influences that was specifically Peruvian. Mariátegui was an advocate for a Marxist-based land reform, whereby nationalism would be expressed in indigenous rural cultures and their labor. Vargas Llosa, in contrast, configures the mixed-blood as a primitive who, on the international level, needs to be subsumed in a broader market integration.

The role femininity plays in mapping the symbolic spaces of civilization, order, economic liberalization, eroticism, and the rationalization of government in Vargas Llosa's work has gone largely unnoticed. In the summer of 1995, when I visited feminist organizations in Lima (Flora Tristán, El

Centro de Documentación sobre la Mujer [Cendoc], and Manuela Ramos), inquiring for information or critique on Vargas Llosa, either his politics or his literary work, from a feminist perspective, the general response was, "You're in the wrong place. We do feminism here," or, simply, if I pressed, "Why?" Most Peruvians I talked to could not tell me what Vargas Llosa's position on women had been. Maruja Barrig recommended that since women were simply containers for class ideology and markers of class interest,[13] and since lesbianism was not featured in any of his novels, I should focus my study on male homosexuality, which was a prominent motif in the entire corpus. Rosario de Bedoya, the secretary who currently maintains Vargas Llosa's office in San Isidro, when I asked her what women's role would be in Vargas Llosa's vision of national renewal, did a computer search of the archival material. She came up with two articles. One was a manuscript of a speech given by Vargas Llosa in Washington, D.C., in 1994, which investigated what Vargas Llosa observed as the increasing feminization of literature and culture, a tendency toward making it sentimental and mysterious, a tendency that, he said, blurred the high art–low art distinction. The other was an interview by Mari Rodríguez Ichaso, in which Vargas Llosa defined the nonhierarchical distance, the lapse of communication, between a "condición feminina" and a "condición masculina" as "the mystery of attraction." The reason, I would suggest, that a discourse on women was invisible in the political record was that the campaign was concerned primarily, predominantly, and almost obsessively with neoliberal economic reform.[14]

In Vargas Llosa's 1989 outline of his party's goals, the exclusive mention of women, after a slight nod toward the idea of incorporating middle-class women in production and politics,[15] was in his treatment of the soup kitchens, day care, and health care centers that the new government would institute and the campaign was already instituting in *los pueblos jóvenes. Los pueblos jóvenes* are urban villages on the outskirts of Lima. They have been arising spontaneously, sometimes legally and sometimes extralegally, in increasing numbers and demographic concentration since early in the century. For the most part, the inhabitants are migrants from *la sierra* and the Andean regions who have left their homes owing to the rise in economic deprivation. These regions are also often hotbeds of oppositional political organization, action, and resistance.[16] The way women were made economically visible, then, in the campaign was through the reorganization of urban space into domestic units. The middle-class white women who were active in this program, called Acción Solidaria or PAS,[17] participated as paternalistic instigators, going into *los pueblos jóvenes* to hand out food and clothing, to aid in the development of small industry and commercial enterprises, of *clubs de madres* (mothers' clubs), *guarderías infantiles* (kindergartens), *concinas populares* (communal kitchens), and *cunas maternales* (day-care centers). These women, says Vargas Llosa in *A Fish in the Water*, his memoirs of the campaign, "the great majority of them were housewives, from families with moderate to high incomes, who up until then had lived a rather empty and even frivolous life, blind and deaf to the seething volcano that is the Peru of underdevelopment and wretched poverty" (163).[18] This domestication of *los pueblos jóvenes* served to make domestic activity visible as a political action. Middle-class housewives crossed into the public space of the market, their images already linked to the effusive volcanic fire, *las escorias*, the ever-increasing visibility of misery in the urban (Andean) population—the masses of the new Peru in Lima. The split and simultaneous confluence between domesticity's public and private face shaped and situated neoliberal reform on the borders of the city *and* of the home, in domestic arrangements between white women and the migrant populations of *los pueblos jóvenes.*

During the early part of the century, when urban migration began significantly to transform the Limeño landscape, the influx of shantytown dwellers at the city edges was seen by the middle classes in the capital as a threat to health. The perceived lack of family structures among the popular classes, the supposed frequency with which fathers were abandoning their households (Oliart, 76), was thought to create a breeding ground of prostitution and sexually transmittable diseases that would, in turn, contaminate the *criollo* and aristocratic members of the oligarchy. As a result, middle-class women, like their counterparts in the British Purity Campaign of the nineteenth century, went into these zones on a mission of sanitation. Their efforts to "clean up the cholas, the blacks and the Chinese" (Villavicencio, 177), were slotted as a moral imperative, an attempt through the containment of sex to clean and cure race by whitening it. *Los pueblos jóvenes* were to be sanitized and contained within a domestic organization that would facilitate their convergence into the order of the market.

Throughout the campaign, *los pueblos jóvenes* served as the central model for the economic rejuvenation that was to take place in the new Peru. Vargas Llosa based his economic plan on the researches that Hernando de Soto, founder and director of Peru's Institute for Liberty and Reform, published in *El otro Sendero* (1986).[19] De Soto had found that these informal sectors should be the locus where entrepreneurial creativity could best germinate but that their productivity was significantly curtailed by legal and bureaucratic red tape. De Soto began his study by describing how, during the course of the twentieth century, the masses of migrants into the city had distorted market stability by forming a zone of extralegality. The economic relationships in this zone were based on pure capitalism, unfettered by regulations. Here had surged economic individualism, new enterprise, vertical mobility, mass consumerism, and entrepreneurial creativity. The problem that de Soto observed in this set-up was that the arbitrary enactment of state disciplinary measures could, at any moment, end up clamping down on the merchants, and the merchants would have to relocate. As a result, very little private investment went into these small commercial ventures. Both supply and productivity were sacrificed to a greater mobility, a disorder, a rebellious movement of capital. De Soto's solution was to cut back the bureaucratic delays and procedural obstacles that made access to legal protection impossible for these informal small businesses, allowing free capitalism to grow and develop outside legal constraint. In the prologue to de Soto's book, Vargas Llosa terms this liberalizing revolution of the informal sectors "la libertad": "It is going forward, made reality by an army of victims of the ruling system, who, upon rebelling against it in name of the right to work and to life, discovered the benefits of liberty" (xxix).

The formalizing of these informal sectors was supposed to bring about a civilizing of the economy. That would open the domestic market to foreign investment and productive creativity by integrating the resistance of capitalism itself—its excess—into an expansionist agenda. In the party plan, Vargas Llosa presents his proposal for economic liberalization as a battle being waged against, simultaneously, promiscuity and barbarism:

> With work and tenacity, the Peruvian man conquered it all: he civilized the summits [feminine noun], sowing them and urbanizing them, and he made the tree, the weaving, the village and the rites of living together sprout up

> over the sand. A vast civilizing and tolerant empire, multiple and, in terms of its epoch, modern, surged up where before there had been desolation, promiscuity and barbarism. (5)

Resistant nature needs to be brought into the economic circuit, just as, Vargas Llosa proclaims, the migrants need to be brought into the cities and led into the domestic productive control of the globalized free market—just as Canudos needed to be leveled and tamed, just as the Baroness needed to be freed from archaic patriarchal controls. In contrast to Canudos, where "equally to sexual promiscuity, Canudos has established promiscuous properties: everything belongs to everybody" (60), for the Sebastianas, a new and modern Peru would dominate nature through a technological and imperial organization of property and labor controlled through private management for global production.

Through Sebastiana, Vargas Llosa is shaping Bataille's theory of eroticism into an exploration of the border, conjoining civilization and barbarism, so prevalent in the Latin American tradition of nationalist identity and literary formation.[20] Sebastiana the *macuma*, as the informal "*hueco*," the infertile "*abismo*" that opens the desire for a national literature, represents, like the migrant populations of the urban poor, the internal resistance inviting a formal narrative of the nation as opening up to a global economy. Invoking geographic displacement and migrant economies, the servant Sebastiana, the mixed-blood woman, veils and unveils the very racial histories in which the nation is imagined as surpassing the economic limitations of archaic institutions, isolation, and lawless resistance. She is at the very core of capital's desires for unbounded market expansion, for excess, and for the economy's lawless resistance to the state's authoritarian controls as it moves toward privatization.

The Rainforest Rape

In order to renew this tender pact between belly and nature, a rotting forest offers its deceptive latrines. . . . An Englishwoman, transfigured by a halo of blond hair, abandons her splendid body to the lubricity and the imagination (driven to the point of ecstasy by the stunning odor of decay) of a number of nude men. . . .

Above the entwined human beasts who embrace and handle her, she raises her marvelous head, so heavy with dazzlement, and her eyes open on a scene of madness.

—Georges Bataille, "The Pineal Eye"

The fantasy world is not unlike the nature reserves which are set up to preserve the original natural state of the country.

—Laplanche and Pontalis, "Fantasy and the Origins of Sexuality"

In fact only a few basic stories are told, over and over, about Native Americans and other "tribal" peoples. These societies are always either dying or surviving, assimilating or resisting. Caught between a local past and a global future, they either hold on to their separateness or "enter the modern world." The latter entry—tragic or triumphant—is always a step toward a global future defined by technological progress, national and international cultural relations. Are there other possible stories?

—James Clifford, *The Predicament of Culture*

On Sunday, 31 May 1992, Paulinho Paiakan, the world-renowned environmentalist activist of the Kaiapó in Brazil, allegedly raped and mutilated, and then attempted to strangle with barbed wire the seventeen-year-old white schoolgirl Silvia Letícia da Luz Ferreira, Paiakan's next-door neighbor and the baby-sitter and tutor of his children.[1] Rob Buchanan, a correspondent for *Details* magazine, reports that "the girl claimed that after actively assisting her husband's aggression, Irekran [Paiakan's wife] had raped her again, putting her hands together in the shape of a cone and penetrating her until 'something tore'" (47).[2]

On 10 June, Brazil's weekly newspaper *Veja*[3] headlined the story "EXPLOSION OF SAVAGE INSTINCT" ("A explosão do instinto selvagem").[4] The article quoted José Barbosa de Souza, the sheriff of Redenção—who, two days after the assault, found the car where the rape had occurred—as saying, "It [the car] was covered with blood from floor to ceiling. It looked like an animal had been slaughtered there" (Buchanan, 47).[5] *Veja* reports a delegate from the hospital where Ferreira was examined as commenting, "The exams proved that there was violence and cannibalistic acts that one would have thought didn't exist anymore" (69). The affidavits, collected and prepared by the sheriff with the assistance of a doctor from the hospital, described the event, according to *Veja*, as "a demonic ritual." In the documents, Ferreira testifies, "'They threaded their two hands into me, like they wanted to scratch everything.' With hands soiled in blood, Irekran went on to smear her body and that of her husband" (71).

Responding against foreign solidarity's defense of Paiakan, *Veja* rejoined: "[Paiakan] symbolized the modern Hollywood version of the Indian: the ideal savage, full of ancestral knowledge, virtuous in his ecological universe—primitive and perfect. Unfortunately, this is only a reinvention of the Indian, as false as the savage portrayed in the John Wayne films as the cruel redskin, always ready to scalp the white man" (Buchanan, 48).[6] As the case moved through trial, Carlos Amaury Azevedo, Paiakan's FUNAI (Fundação Nacional do Indio) defense lawyer, contended that "it was Irekran alone who had perpetrated the attack" (Buchanan, 53).[7]

The same week (3–14 June), the Earth Summit took place in Rio de Janiero.[8] Meanwhile, the president of Brazil, Fernando Collor de Mello, was under investigation on charges of extortion and corruption for which he would later be forced to resign from office. As the federal crisis was being exposed in the media, P. C. Farias, "the man behind the huge network of corruption and profiteering underlying the Collor presidency, also exposed during the Rio conference," was portrayed in Brazil's *Veja* with "the addition of a feather headdress" (McCallum, 5). It was also revealed that Collor's wife was complicit in dipping her hands into the state treasury. The Paiakan rape case exposes the nation, Cecilia McCallum concludes, as "relegate[d] . . . forever to the murky depths of savagery" (19).

The crisis in federal authority and credibility was partly attributed to Collor's Indian policies. Having campaigned as the "environmental president," Collor had set up national reserves on indigenous territories, measuring them and mapping them in order to regulate the application of Indian law, the preservation of customs, the trade in timber and valuable minerals, and contingently, the sustainable development of natural resources in the Amazon region.[9] In November 1991, Collor set aside 36,000 square miles for the Yanomama. He also approved reserving 42,471 square miles for the Kaiapó (see Whittemore, 7). The *Veja* article, however, complains that the federal mandate to reserve territories was not funded, and so the Brazilian Air Force could not adequately enforce the policy (see 73). The lines of demarcation that set off Indians on their lands were therefore constantly being illegally infringed upon by speculators in valuable minerals.

What this event revolves around is a general sense on the part of the environmentalist movement, government, and corporate interests alike that nature is outside the culture of capital. David Harvey has shown how current rhetoric describing a planetary state of ecological crisis has tended to coalesce around this issue, allowing for working alliances between corporate capitalism and green politics. As nature is endangered by social forces, the argument goes, it is in need of dire technological interventions and increased management to protect it from universal devastation. Management would include increasing practices of efficiency, productivity, and conservation, practices that would ease the possibilities of accumulation and the extension of the resource base. Such environmentalist responses are, says Harvey, "compatible with a segment of corporate capital's concerns to rationalize planetary management of the world's global resources in the name of ecological modernization" (329).

In addition, this position exhibits a major difference for program implementation between rich and poor nations; it divides initiatives for economic *development* from distinctive measures for economic *growth*. Technologically advanced countries are presented as the problem solvers, whereas other countries are positioned as the problems themselves, the part that needs to be managed through the increasingly hard-handed grip of corporate and federal controls. We have all heard news stories, for instance, about how the overpopulation of the Third World is causing environmental depletion and so such countries are in need of population control measures. These same stories, however, neglect to mention the role of multinational industry, a role that would seem more crucial to consider given the comparative amount of pollutants and damage emitted. This configuration of responsibility not only excuses interventions that pave the way for capitalist expansion and fuller market integration but also mask a fundamentally racist agenda whereby nonwhite peoples are, time and again, assumed to be helpless children in need of paternalistic, corporate advice, assistance, and discipline.

The Paiakan case exhibits another dimension of situating environmental crisis as a struggle between a resolute nature and its fatherly management. Harvey was not wrong in remarking the romanticization of nature, in environmentalist discourse, as being outside the social, when in actuality the production of nature is always *inside* of historical movements of capital. He gives the example of highways and cityscapes, which produce their own ecosystems contingent to and dependent on capital dispersements. This contingency is exactly what the Paiakan case makes visible; it is just like what is depicted in the extensive news coverage of natural disasters—hurricanes, floods, forest fires. Not even the most devoted efforts of firefighters or the national guard, nor the most doting visits and speeches of the vice president, nor the most sincere edicts of the president can save us from catastrophe. Millions are made homeless, their property and crops destroyed. The difference in the Paiakan story is that it reveals how capital rather than nature has become too free, overflowing its barriers, its challenge too fierce; capital itself has taken on the role of the undisciplined.

Paiakan symbolizes the collapse between nature and capital or, rather, the naturalization of global capitalist competition at an extreme. The unruly Indian is the purveyor of cruel capital, performing criminal acts that demand a more benevolent side of capital to step in. In a sense, Paiakan's story is the story of success. It tells of a people who have successfully negotiated a position within media networks and worked out their own corporate profit sectors. The Kaiapó have, in fact, been "recognized" in that vital sense of the term: they have framed their own subjectivities and become political agents within a postcolonial power contest and have, as well, acquired the means to control their own representations. Thomas Friedman described them as a case of successful globalization. Citing Glenn Prickett, senior vice-president of Conservation International, Friedman attests,

> The Kayapo have defended a large chunk of intact Amazon for centuries through sheer force. Now they are learning to protect it through alliances with international scientists, conservationists and socially conscious business people.... While sitting in this hut with the leading men of the village, I noticed that they were all watching a single TV, connected to a large satellite dish. The men were flipping the channels back and forth between a Brazilian soccer match and a business channel that carried the running price of gold on world markets.... [The Kayapo men] used [the] profits earned on the world gold market to protect their own unique lifestyle in the middle of the Amazon rain forest. (30–31)

What is "successful" about the Kaiapó is the way they exemplify the success of the market, proving that it is the equalizer in even the most exotic of settings. Friedman is unable to grasp that the price of this "success" is not the protection of unique lifestyles but rather the universal adoption, as the scene makes clear, of cultures of capital and consumption and the ability to reduce all cultures to profit motivations within a system of universal exchangeability and commodification.

In the Paiakan rape story, however, an image of corporate caring is promoted, one that precludes any agenda for racial justice or cultural diversity by linking Third World competition to murderous, rapacious impulses. Paiakan remains in the position of embodying the uncontrollable revenge of nature in need of corporate adjustments, a type of primitive capitalism making "partnerships" to promote a greater consumerism. As Thomas Friedman says, "If you want to save the Amazon, go to business school and learn how to do a deal" (229). Neoliberal doctrine says free markets are the answer to economic and social problems. So to expand economies globally, the best course of action is to lower trade barriers and privatize. However, neoliberalism benefits from protectionism in the form of state subsidies that prop up private industry or even state actions, like the Asian bailout, which set up economic infrastructures benefiting transnational corporations and finance over domestic production in the name of "market discipline." As Noam Chomsky observes, "One fundamental component of free trade theory is that public subsidies are not allowed. But after World War II, U.S. business leaders expected that the economy would head right back to depression without state intervention" (36). Brazil's protections of indigenous lands and rights obstruct labor's speculation in timber, gold, and markets while opening up access to transnational corporations through contracting. Chomsky continues, "The problem of Latin America is not 'populism,' Brazilian economist Bresser Pereira points out, but 'subjection of the state to the rich.'" ... Even the World Bank concedes that foreign investment and the privatization it hails 'has tended to substitute for other capital flows' in Latin America, transferring control and sending profits abroad" (33). Paiakan's story exhibits the excess of capital's invisible hand.

The recognition of the Kaiapó coincides with a neoliberalization of the Brazilian economy in the wake of the military dictatorships ending in 1985. As Edward Herman and Robert McChesney have shown, Brazilian media monopolization was rewarded by the generals in the form of large state subsidies, advertising contracts, satellite support, and the like, the very technologies that allow Friedman to see the Kaiapó as proving global capital's embrace of diversity. The civilian administrators who followed did not intervene in the consolidation of the media, and as a result, the media were instrumental in supporting Collor's candidacy and his neoliberal platform over his left-wing opponent favored by labor. The weekly magazine *Veja*, where the Paiakan story broke, is part of the vast *O Globo* empire supporting the opening up of the Brazilian economy to foreign investments and the concentration of the economy under large-scale corporate control, thus helping to establish huge economic inequalities. Herman and McChesney point out that the recognition of marginal cultures demonstrates

> the liberalizing effects of the coming of TV in remote Brazilian villages, hungry of contacts with the outside world and influenced by more progressive (feminist, anti-authoritarian) perspectives coming from the urban centers. At the same time, there is an isolating effect, a new individualist and consumerist ideology that begins to take hold.... This form was capable of incorporating traditional oral folk cultures, but these were ultimately structured with the dominant themes being "upward mobility and consumer consumption." ... This system of positive messages, uplift, and evasion of political issues was just what the military dictatorship and advertising community wanted; it protected a system of immense inequality, helped to keep

> the public diverted, the public sphere shriveled and subtly biased, and inculcating values that keep people isolated and depoliticized. . . . In our view, the most important fact about *Globo* and the media system in place in Brazil is that it is advertisement-based and part of a global system that will press consumerist and neoliberal ideology, unremittingly and with vast resources. (166)

The Kaiapó success in controlling timber and gold markets and owning property as well as their involvement in media is certainly a tale of uplift; it suggests that capitalism promotes freedom and democratizes access to profits and production. The Paiakan case projected a neoliberal vision of a universal embrace of diverse cultures but then showed these cultures to be at fault for social conflict. What never entered the discussion was how the conflict between a poor, white, rural population and a capitalist class composed of a few indigenous exemplars was the result of large corporations limiting people's power over and access to their economic futures. The conflict in the story is not shown as a struggle between classes for control over resources or as a challenge to the corporate agenda. Rather, it is presented cinemagraphically as a war in which cultural difference stands in for individual autonomy, the right to consume, and the right to profit by exploiting other people's labor.

Embedded in this scenario, too, is the idea that women, rather than markets, are up for grabs in the intensifying crossfire of deregulated competition. There is definitely a sense here that the patriarchal family has weakened, leaving women open to the seductive allures of the new capitalist class. The contention of who is in control of women's sexuality turns into the question of who commands the markets. The desire to consume fits the popular media into a narrative about women's sexuality no longer under the tight scrutiny of paternalistic regulation.

Collor's land reforms were implemented through unbalanced paternalistic state interventions into isolated communities under protectionist policies. The state was to be the guardian of Indians who, territorially separated, were outside of national market integration, standing in for Indian interests in juridical and economic controversies. Based on the tenet that Indians were *"relativamente incapaces"* (relatively incapable) (Carneiro da Cunha, 28), this *titulado* system, originating in the 1916 Civil Code and presently under the jurisdiction of FUNAI, where Paiakan had worked as a representative, was at the time under contention in Brazilian politics because of the increasing difficulty of thinking of the Indian as isolated and nonassimilated.[10] Also, changes in the Indian statues in 1983 allowed the government to grant mining concessions even on demarcated lands, thereby harnessing more power to neoliberal agendas and marking an end to the military regimes.

The constitutional definition of the Indian in Brazil is based mostly on territory, ancestry, a consciousness of historical continuity with a pre-Columbian past, and the practice of traditions, such as rituals. A category for "integrados," that is, Indians "incorporated in the national community and recognized in full exercise of civic rights, but who conserve the uses, costumes and traditions characteristic of their culture" (Carneiro da Cunha, 23), was being considered on the national level.[11] In this extensively debated controversy, Paiakan's Indianness was put into doubt because of his wealth and his contacts with international environmental activist groups. The anthropologist Cecilia McCallum commented:

> Was it not the case that as tutees of the State and "relatively incapable" they could not be prosecuted? But Payakan was a rich, property-owning, car-driving, voting Indian. No longer a real Indian at all in fact, it was alleged. The debate focused increasingly upon the bastardization of Kayapo culture. In the space of twenty years, from the time they had supposedly been "first contacted" by white men, their materialism and alliances with international interests had led them to lose their culture. Payakan (like many of Brazil's newly "false" Indians) could be prosecuted. (5–6)

The ambiguities of Indian identity in the constitutional debates became part of Paiakan's court performance. The prosecuting attorney, Lucia Rosa da Silva, insisted that the court try Paiakan and Irekran as "Brazilians just like the rest of us." Paiakan, she said, was "just another rich man"; he had a driver's license, bank account, and passport, whereas Irekran dressed "like a civilized woman." Yet, Paiakan and Irekran both appeared in court in the full regalia of "Indian": "Paiakan, his chest black and his feet red with war paint, flew out of Aukre accompanied by five small airplanes full of chiefs and warriors.... Brandishing bows and arrows and thick wooden spears, they stormed the streets of Redencao in a convoy of pickup trucks, then formed a blockade in front of the courthouse chanting a rolling war call"

(Preston, 1). And "Irekran, 24, came to the courthouse with her cheeks and arms inked with the stunning black and geometric designs of Kaiapo tradition. She ... had shaved a triangle across the crown of her head, as Kaiapo women do" (Preston). The courthouse and rape trial became a stage for the full-fledged display of savagery and Kaiapó nonassimilation.[12]

This story—about an indigenous activist who crosses a cultural border by participating in global market transactions, to create a specifically "local" representation of political involvement—emerges through a narrative of interracial rape.[13] In the Brazilian popular media's reports on the case, free-flowing and uninhibited markets, capital, and profit came to be positioned as a visibly oppositional and transformative sign of assimilation and the loss of "Indianness." Writes, for example, Francisco Viana in *Isto É*, "European ecologists now find that business deals transformed Paiakan into a man of great power and richness, bringing about, as a consequence, 'the corruption and alienation of indigenous culture'" (38). Inside these representations are embedded assumptions about how "real Indians" do not make contracts with mining interests, timber companies, or cosmetic firms; do not own airplanes and trucks; and do not speak English and Portuguese. That is, "real Indians" are not "*bons capitalistas.*" "Independent of how much they squander with their typical customs of nouveau-riches," reports Viana, "which include their constant flights to the city to buy bananas, for example, the Indians already represent a respectable economic potency, and are in permanent ascent" (40). Contingent to these underlying messages, interracial sex is imagined as a product of such "savage capital" (40). Viana goes on to state, "Conjugal unions between whites and Indians are not part of the local customs, but one night of love could bring [the white prostitutes] payments of around US $100" (92).

The assuming of Indianness that the constitutional ambiguity demanded took place as a staging of a stereotype, a mobilization of an available repertoire of imagery defining ethnicity, the fetish in which is contained, as Homi Bhabha expounds in "The Other Question," "a space for a 'subject peoples' through the production of knowledges" where the social reality of the "other" is bounded within a "recognizable totality" both "knowable and visible" (316). Because the legal definition of Indian identity centered on the visibility of custom and tradition, the constitutional battle and the entire cultural politics in which the Kaiapó were engaged was waged on the level of the image, on the performance of Indianness. In the past twenty years or so, ever since the Kaiapó were systematically integrated into the Brazilian national economy when gold and mahogany were discovered on their territories, the Kaiapó have increasingly structured their ethnic identity around a politics of visibility. By means of interventions with media, the Kaiapó have repeatedly produced a separate and marginal ethnic identity for themselves through, paradoxically, their increasing involvement with strategies of Western technological imaging. Notes anthropologist Terence Turner: "The use of video media to represent themselves and other indigenous people as distinct social and political entities defined by distinct 'cultures,' in other words, was very probably one of the major influences responsible for the Kayapos' development of their new conception of 'Kayapo culture'" ("Social Dynamics," 70). During the 1970s, journalists, anthropologists, and international support groups introduced video recording equipment to the Kaiapó.[14] By the late 1970s, remarks Turner, a major figure in the implementation and development of indigenous media among the Kaiapó, "these visitors made the Kayapo aware that the outside world, beyond the limited circle of local Brazilian frontier society and national government officials, values their culture and was generally inclined to support their political and land rights" ("Visual Media," 34). In 1985, Brazilian researchers donated a camcorder, a videocassette recorder deck, and a monitor to the Kaiapó community of Gorotire. In 1987 and again in 1989, Turner, consulting on documentaries about the Kaiapó for Granada's *Disappearing World* series, left behind more camcorders, tapes, monitors, a VCR, and batteries in appreciation for the Kaiapós' cooperation. He subsequently arranged and organized, with the aid of Vincent Carelli and the Centro de Trabalho Indigenista (CTI), training, editing, and storage projects in São Paulo, where the more advanced facilities and more temperate climate allowed for the tapes to be better preserved. Remarks Turner, "The Kayapo have used their own capacity for video in a variety of ways: the documentation of their own traditional culture, above all ceremonial performances; secondly, the recording of important events . . . ; and thirdly, as an organizing tool" (34).[15]

The irony of the Kaiapós' use of video equipment is that it visualizes an authentic culture of difference and opposition only through technologies of capital. The Kaiapós' involvement with technology actually came up in the court trial as a point that was to prove that the Indians were assimilated into white culture, and so not really Indians at all:

> JUDGE: "I understand that you know how to operate a VCR. Is this true?"
> PAYAKAN: "Yes, Your Honor."
> JUDGE: "How can you call yourself an Indian if you work with these machines? Even I don't know how to use a VCR. How can you be a real Indian?"
> PAYAKAN: "Your Honor, the only reason that I know how to operate a VCR and your Honor doesn't is because I took the time to learn." (Conklin, 715)

Part of the construction of the Kaiapó culture of visibility is the visibility of the native cinematographer, the concrete exposure of the Kaiapó gaze, within that frame. "Kayapo culture" is thus formulated as what can be seen of what the Kaiapó see: a culture that is constantly consuming inasmuch as it becomes the object of consumption.[16] Constructing Kaiapó ceremonial structure as its own cinemagraphability, the film *The Kayapo Out of the Forest* cuts regularly to images of long-haired Indians, mostly on the margins of the frame, with one eye buried in the viewer of hand-held video cameras. The film moves from viewing the roving Indian with the camera to viewing and becoming the view itself, allowing the Indian with the camera to be what orients and controls the image in which he is also embedded or, as James Clifford puts it, "a state of being in culture while looking at culture" (9).

The insistent returning to this image of the Kaiapó—with long hair and war paint—arrayed with technological equipment, places the idea of their survival on the world stage, making visible how capitalist power is causing nature and cultures of difference to appear as if they are disappearing. Fatimah Tobing Rony has discussed how ethnographic film creates moments of eternal repetition to counterbalance "the native"'s eternal return (as in Eliade's conception of myth) against the flow of time, history, and progress: "As intended . . . , this form of ethnographic film, infused with the notion of death and the idea of vanishing races, is a cinema of archetypal moments endlessly repeated" (102). The idea, operational in Turner's explications of indigenous media, that culture can be exhausted on a visual plane, that the visual plane actually stands for what culture is by definition and in whole, simplistically assumes that cultural experience can be reduced to its image, and that imagery in turn assures cultural endurance against what is professed as its imminent extinction and the disappearance of the forest.

The Kaiapó's camera gaze is used here as a technique of recognition but also as a tool that recognizes a disappearance. In Freud, the gaze works within the castration narrative to explain the ways the psyche develops through the threat of disappearance. The little boy notices that his sister or his mother does not have the organ that he has and becomes obsessed with the threat that his, too, will disappear. In film theory, this same gaze produces gendered identification. For example, women, Laura Mulvey (1975) says, represent the "to-be-looked-at-ness" of the image, creating the recognition of difference and the possibility of subjectivity—of self-preservation, a defense against disappearance—in the voyeurism of the (male) spectator. As long as the woman is there to be looked at in pictures, the logic goes, all cannot be lost. In the Kaiapó case, however, what is threatening to disappear is the forest itself. Psychoanalysis presupposes a psyche devoid of history and economic interests. In contrast, the Kaiapó story shows how disappearance is not merely a matter of shifting eyes and cinematic identifications. Rather, the very visible disappearance of Kaiapó culture makes the Kaiapó into a commodity.

Conceiving Kaiapó culture as the image, like the Barthian photograph, of a reality disappearing raises many issues in thinking through the relationships between essence and image, between culture and visibility, between recognition and politics, between resistance and representation, between ethnographic film and the "ethnicities" supposed to be contained in it. Here the image of disappearance is what creates cultural difference, posing the question of whether recognition is enough of a criterion for political agenda-setting, whether identity politics can be based on something besides recognition. For Terry Turner, as for Barthes, authenticity and difference are acts of repetition whose referent begins to exist, to appear, at the moment of its repetition, of its placement as past, as disappearing. Writing retrospectively about his first encounter with the Kaiapó of Gorotire in 1962, Turner discusses how the transformations to Kaiapó cultural practice as a result of interaction with missionaries were only surface deep. Underneath a thin veneer of concrete social changes in the "outward forms of

Kayapo life and culture," "the authentic Kayapo culture still persisted" ("Representing, Resisting," 291), discernible by and redeemable through the anthropologist's trained eye. The authenticity of Kaiapó culture, which Turner claims to have seen beneath the cover of missionary impositions and assimilationalist social rearrangements, is precisely a culture defined as its own visibility:

> Although the Gorotire themselves had given us a friendly welcome, we[17] were depressed, upset, and confused, even more by Gorotire's failure to live up to our idea of what a Kayapo village should look like than by the *encarregado*'s hostile reception. As we gloomily considered our situation, women, girls, and a few men began to assemble at one side of the street near the men's house. They were nude, their bodies painted and covered between the knees and the neck with parakeet feathers, their cheeks decorated with crushed blue eggshell stuck on with resin, their earlobes distended with large mother-of-pearl earrings made of freshwater mussel shells, and their torsos hung with ornamental sashes and baby-slings. (289)

The entire reading of what authentic culture is, Turner insinuates, reduced to the ceremony, where dancing, circling native bodies divest themselves of Western "shorts and occasionally T-shirts" to reveal the truth of their nudity, ritual ornaments, and scarification.[18] The ceremony, ethnicity, marginality, and cultural identity all constitute, in this passage, the real to be retrieved or recovered in the anthropological engagement with the Kaiapó.

The ceremony where Turner, in 1962, gets his first glimpse of an authentic "Kayapo culture" and then, where "Kayapo culture" reappears beneath the "overlay" of its disappearance in assimilation, ends in a ritual performance of cultural origins in rape. Cultural difference emerges specifically through a violent (Turner suggests "playful") re-enactment of "Kayapo culture," the moment of cultural defense from conquest and assimilation constituted through women's revenge: "As the sun finally rose over the exhausted column of dancers, armed men suddenly appeared and began seizing girls and women from the line.... As they raced away, dragging their captives towards the houses, they were pursued by older women ..., who brandished burning logs, with which they beat the backs of the retreating warriors" (291).

Turner's framing of culture as the visible fashions culture itself into a figure of resistance ("Representing, Resisting," 294).[19] He asserts that the persistence of ceremony is not a mode of accommodation with "imposed political, social, and ideological forms constituting the situation of contact" (292) but instead a strategy for a culture of redemption. Likewise, in some postcolonial theoretical literature, the Kaiapó video project is discussed variously as an example of the privileged decentering of "polycentric multiculturalism," a disruptive decentering in that it brings into relief cultural relativism (Stam, 117–18), or a paradigm for resistance demonstrating how a "cultural hybridity and a capacity for mimicry" and "a strategic requirement to recover . . . a past" can be used for "preserving the essential contours of their culture" (Shohat, 175). Certainly, however, the rise of Kaiapó video is not simply a typical example of an "oppressed peoples" claiming rights and recognition in the face of hegemonic reprisals. The successful mediation of Kaiapó wealth and position in institutional networks is done in part through a strategic construction of visibility as a discourse on survival, continuity, environmental crisis, oppositional identity, and representational disappearance. Should the Kaiapó project of prospecting in valuable minerals and timber and acquiring landed properties be judged on different terms and by different criteria than enterprises more easily labeled, perhaps, as multinational and/or consumer capitalism? Does their symbolic status as "redeemers" and "protectors" let the Kaiapó off the hook, so to speak, or is it the only or the best way for indigenous peoples in a global context to assume powers of communication and viable political clout? Is assimilation into the global capitalist order really the only way to imagine resistance and redemption?

Rachel Moore criticizes indigenous video, and the Kaiapó project in particular, for fashioning the visible, in its play on the margins, as a fictive recuperation of the real, "a fetish," thus reproducing the assumptions underlying traditional (Western) representational practices and their status as commodities. For Moore, such core structural implications as "the burden of representation," "the authority of the camera itself" (17), "the authenticity of the native's voice," the positivistic appeal of science as a record of reality (18), and the containment of population within a surveillable space (19) all work to rearticulate a scientific rationalism that shores up anthropology's investment in the mythologies of realism with its conscription and collection of "the margins." The Indian as a visible entity reproduces itself as the plasticity of the center. The postion that the culture of the image is also a token sign of cultural resistance, or a technique for preserving the material reality of a disappearing people, or a privileged site for a decentered postcolonial politics of speech, or a form of cultural recognition and an expression of cultural diversity, is not so simply assumed.

Within Kaiapó cultural politics, disappearance is the central trope through which Kaiapó culture is visualized as a culture of redemption. Yet, how does disappearance become a subject of film? Luce Irigaray's work might be useful here, for the positioning of the feminine as the threat of disappearance is linked in her work to anxieties of economic dissipation. The image stores, collects, and preserves material acquisitions against possible dissolution into the feminine. "If what you want to get hold of, keep, accumulate, is perishable," she says, "if one look, for example, can change its value, then the toil and the war will be relentless and endless" (95). The image is therefore organized as a fetish and repeated as a mask for the threatened domination of the overdetermined visible signifier of masculinity and power. In her readings of Freud's philosophic presumptions, the fetish, the imperative to a repetition, an overdetermination of the real, of the visible, guards against the material disappearance that the feminine assures.

In the Kaiapó case, the imaging of culture exhibits the breaking down of territories. In turn, such territories are drawn and defended in narratives of marriageability, family, and reproduction. In the Kaiapó-directed film *Peace between Chiefs,* the controversy that the chiefs debate centers on a dispute over a community's hunting and gathering incursions in another community's legal range of economic activity and profit. The usual method, in the past, for the Kaiapó to resolve conflicts was through "village fission" (Bamberger, 133); that is, a party would split off from the community to set up residence somewhere else. This "fission" has spread the territory the Kaiapó would inhabit and has become a problem for national policy makers who want to circumscribe an exclusive juridical area for native economic activity and the rational application of land, environmental, and indigenous rights. Actually, as Rachel Moore has argued, the containment of the Kaiapó within a fixed boundary is "something new to them which accommodates the Brazilian state's need to contain the population" (19). But the politics of vision that enclose Kaiapó culture are also stabilized within familial boundaries. The conflict is resolved when Chief Raoni announces that they should all go home, at which point they board airplanes that take them out of the circumscribed reach of the camera. Beyond the place of the meeting delineated in the lens are the wives through whom the chiefs reference the territories in question. "Chiefs should not make passes at their followers' wives," Chief Raoni proclaims, meaning that they should only hunt within their own territory. Sex marks the private ownership of territory.

The film's closure in marriage furnishes a way of quite literally grounding the image in the cultured space of market normalization symbolized through the family.[20]

In *Veja*'s telling, the defense of the virgin forest *(mata virgem)* is, in fact, connected to the defense of the Brazilian family as a means, says a letter to the editors of the *New York Times*, to "prevent the destruction of their natural patrimony." The story in *Veja* starts by showing the rape as resulting from a lapse in Ferreira's paternal surveillance. Leticia, the article remarks, lives with her parents and eleven siblings and goes to school. What is more, "She doesn't have a boyfriend and she was a virgin, as the doctors ... have proved" (69). In fact, Ferreira's virginity—a reminder of paternal surveillance—becomes the focus of the rape charge, putting paternal control over female sexuality at the center of the defense's concerns. "She [Irekran] hurled vindictives at Ferreira," observes Scott Wallace in a *Penthouse* article, "challenging the plaintiff's claim that she'd lost her virginity that night to Paiakan. 'I want her to look me in the face and tell me she was a virgin,' Irekran sneered" (109). The rape occurred, *Veja* continues, when Leticia's parents were spending the weekend on a farm fifty miles outside of Redenção, leaving Leticia alone in town with her 12-year-old sister and a girlfriend from school. According to *Veja,* the temporary loosening of familial control corresponds to Leticia's friendship with "da família do cacique" (the family of the chief); in the parents' absence, Paiakan went to her house to invite her to the barbecue where the rape would take place. Waldemir Ferriera, Leticia's father, interpreted the rape, according to Julia Preston of the *Washington Post,* as an affront to familial honor that could only be reclaimed through the reinstatement of paternal authority: "'He's international, he's rich, but this time he tangled with a family that is poor but respectable,' said Waldemir Ferreira, the victim's father, a farmer with a broad-rimmed cowboy hat. He patted the place on his belt where he hooks his pistol when he decides to carry it. 'If the court doesn't make him pay, I will face him man to man to collect my debt.'" The lack of vigilance on the part of the father leaves the white woman open to indigenous control of her heredity, just as the weakening of federal authority leaves the forest open to confiscation by Indian economic interests.

The domestic component of Kaiapó identity contributed to the legislating of land reforms. The figuring of land in the film *Peace between Chiefs* (produced by Terence Turner in collaboration with the Kaiapó) works to insinuate a politics of family settlement and stationariness as the basis for preserving Kaiapó culture. The film ends with the union of husband and wife, just as in movie Westerns, Laura Mulvey argues, the themes of marriage and homestead most often finalize the plot. Themes of marriage and homestead, says Mulvey, "transform the terrain of adventure and discovery into a land in which settlement, and consequently the sphere of the feminine, can be established" (1992: 56).[21] Specifically, Paiakan has been represented as a hero of the environmental cause, battling villains, polluters, land developers, miners, loggers, rugged adventurers, and the Brazilian government, in the name of defending, protecting, and finally winning, for his culture, the virgin forest. Against all odds, against opposition and conspiracy within the Kaiapó communities themselves, in defiance of the growing desire for money instigated by an influx of consumer products, Paiakan alone, the story goes, held out, not wanting to sell the timber rights, resisting the loggers' lucrative offers of material goods in the hopes of "preserving the forest." In Rob Buchanan's article, Paiakan is depicted as a hero defending domesticity in the face of an aggressive culture of adventurism and profiteering. The warrior Paiakan, at "the threshold of Brazil's wild west" (46), on the border of "a typical Brazilian boomtown with cash machines and Chevy pick-ups and gunplay in the afternoon" (48), is photographed standing with a gun in front of his house and car, Irekran and his three daughters scattered around him.

Savagery, as excess desire, surges out of the irresistible temptation offered in the white commodity world, which would make Kaiapó culture disappear. "An investigation by the environmental group, Friends of the Earth," contends the *Wall Street Journal*, "found that Kayapo chiefs . . . have allowed loggers to extract at least 40,000 cubic yards of mahogany—about 1,500 truckloads—in exchange for an airplane, motor vehicles and some Western-style houses." The difficulties brought to bear on Kaiapó culture through excessive capital consumption become health problems. Continues the *Journal:* "Chief [Tutu] Pombo ... took the lead among Kayapo chieftains who made deals with developers. By 1990, the chief, whose net worth was estimated at $6 million, owned three ranches, several cars and an airplane with his likeness painted on the fuselage. When Tutu Pombo died of hypertension two years later, his doctors laid part of the blame on the chief's predilection for 'white man's food,' chocolate and sugar."[22] Paiakan himself started making contracts with the loggers in 1990. In 1989 he started extracting oils from Brazil nuts that were to be sold to The Body Shop, a multinational corporation, for hair conditioner. In the logic of these stories, the Kaiapó desire for commodities threatens the reproduction of their culture. In *Veja*, there is a photograph of a logging truck being loaded by Kaiapó men. The caption reads: "Wood extracted from the reserve: 60 millions of dollars for the Kaiapó." Opposite, Paiakan and his family, Irekran and the three girls, are shown dining in a restaurant. The waiter, dressed in a buttoned-down shirt with a bowtie, is carrying abundantly filled plates. The caption reads, "Paiakan in a restaurant with the family: displeasure for not having a son" (73). Thus, Kaiapó assimilation and desire for commodities are figured as an ethnic reproductive problem.

What Irekran is afraid of when she looks at Ferreira's body, she confesses, is that "she [Ferreira] could give Paiakan a son." The day before the incident, she [Irekran] said, she and Ferreira had gone swimming at a waterhole. "She kept telling me that her body was younger and prettier than mine," Irekran said. In the car coming back from the Sunday picnic, "I pretended to be asleep, but I was thinking about what she had said" (Preston).[23] The year before, a doctor in Redencao had tied Irekran's fallopian tubes when she had gone in for an abortion:

> After she suffered a series of life-threatening miscarriages, a white doctor in Redencao operated to prevent her from having new pregnancies. The doctor and a witness said in interviews that Irekran had consented to the operation. But Paiakan was incensed and claimed that, because he needed a son to carry on his family line as a Kaiapo chief, the operation was grounds for him to leave the marriage.... Eventually Irekran denied she had agreed to the

> operation and Paiakan sued the doctor. Both men said that Irekran's "problems in the head" since the surgery accounted for her rage against Ferreira.[24]

Certainly, Irekran's sterilization would signify an alteration in the economic transfer of Kaiapó patrimony. *Veja* notes, "Irekran started to drink a lot ever since she lost her last son, a year ago. Paiakan always wanted to have a son who could succeed him as the tribe's lead. A year ago, his wife had an emergency operation in Redenção. Without consulting anyone, the doctor Ederson da Silva decided to tie the Indian's tubes. There was a tentative mishap in trying to retie the tubes in São Paulo. Besides opening a legal suit against the doctor, Paiakan continued to threaten to separate from his wife in order to marry another woman who could give him the desired son" (70).

However, among the Kaiapó, chieftainship [the position of *ben-iadjuòrò*] is not hereditary, and as Joan Bamberger observes, "the amount of influence each leader has is directly contingent on personal qualities" (138). As for the ancestral blood line, Turner insisted in a telephone interview that this was not a concern in Kaiapó social practice. In his analysis of Kaiapó kinship in "Kinship, Household and Community Structure among the Kayapó," Turner argues that in the Kaiapó "uxorilocal" system, familial attachments and affinities get passed down to the son-in-law, in the wife's natal residence, when he has the children who allow him integration into the wife's family unit. In the phone interview, Turner called Paiakan's statement that he needed a son to pass down the chieftainship "hype for the whiteman." Though Paiakan's father is a *ben-iadjuòrò*, Paiakan himself has never been entitled so among the Kaiapó. In "The Social Dynamics of Video," Turner argues that Paiakan's political leverage was achieved not through the reproduction of the lineage in the son but instead through the possession of the video camera.[25] Kaiapó sterility is equated to being seen seeing, desiring, and then accessing "white" technological cultures of reproduction.

Paiakan, it is said, finally was forced to cave in and make concessions to the capitalism he was seemingly resisting. So, even as he was becoming an internationally recognized environmental activist, he also started making contracts with timber companies. Moreover, the Kaiapó arranged to collect 5 percent of all profits from gold extraction on their territories. The miners themselves lost control when the Kaiapó landed on their airfields dressed as Kaiapó warriors, brandishing weapons. In addition, Paiakan was looking for ways, the story goes, of marrying sustainable development to corporate profits in the name of preserving his culture. In partnership with the British natural cosmetics chain The Body Shop, Paiakan established the first hair conditioner factory in the rain forest. The Body Shop was advertising itself as a corporation with a mission of social justice and featured the Kaiapó on a promotional poster proclaiming, "Trade Not Aid." The company's business arrangements with marginal workers, such as the hiring of orphans in India to manufacture wooden back massagers, were supposed to demonstrate that business was more effective in protecting the poor and ensuring their survival than were relief organizations, international human rights groups, nongovernmental organizations, or global coalitions like the United Nations—that business was fairer, more caring, and more just. There is no evidence, however, that The Body Shop's involvement with the Kaiapó helped any but those few (including Paiakan) in control of production. But the ensuing publicity does suggest rather strongly that the production of culture as a business commodity is the only means for culture to survive. In fact, The Body Shop's presence among the Kaiapó led to rifts, conflicts, and power struggles within the community as well as between communities.

Anita Roddick of The Body Shop, in her self-help guide for "politically aware" entrepreneurs, describes the town of Altamira, the site of the political rally where she first met with Paiakan, as "like something from a very bad Western": "It was a dingy sprawl of shambling single-storey buildings, many of which appeared to be bordellos, with flea-bitten horses tied up outside. The streets were ankle-deep in mud; most of the locals carried guns and looked as if they would be delighted at an excuse to use them" (188–89). Altamira was the site for the 1989 Kaiapó rally convened by Paiakan that would, according to Rob Buchanan's account, "drive a final stake through the heart of" the Xingu Hydroelectric Dam Project (48), the funding for which the Brazilian government was soliciting from the World Bank. In Roddick's description, the lawless border is depicted as a row of buildings exhibiting commercial adventurism through white prostitution.

In opposition, the Kaiapó community at Altamira was, claims Turner, self-consciously imagined as sedentary and domestic: "The encampment of the Kayapo participants was created as a model Kayapo village, complete with families, traditional shelters, and artifact production, all on display for the edification of the hundreds of photo journalists, television and film camera crews, and video cameras" ("Representing, Resisting," 307). The planetary salvation that the Kaiapó as environmentalists promise is represented here as the promise of the family. The line dividing the town and the Kaiapó mock village separates domesticity, sedentariness, and cultural reproduction from sexual labor, circulation, and speculative profit.

Defining the border that separates cultures, white female sexuality is elided into the market economy of the town. Roddick's book encourages business reform through an explicit politics of caring and a return to the feminine,[26] linking commercialism to white femininity. In a full-page color photograph that she inserts in her chapter on the Altamira rally and on her formative Brazil nut contracts with Paiakan, Roddick herself is shown seated on a leafy forestal bed, holding a pen and balancing a notebook on her drawn-up knees. Shadowed by a canopy of lush and deep green vegetation receding into an unfocused distance, the central figure of the white woman is bathed in a burst of light, with a particularly effervescent ring around her head. Surrounding her are two groups of Kaiapó men, partly naked except for beads, feathers, and shorts, one group sitting in front of her, one group standing behind. The caption reads, "Who says we don't have a marketing department?" (195).

In the photograph, the arrangement of figures recalls Edouard Manet's 1863 painting *Le Déjeuner sur l'Herbe*. The white men surrounding the naked white prostitute in the painting are dressed in a somber black, sharpening the effect of the woman's sexuality through color contrast. The front man, reclining on the grass, stretches out an empty hand, as though offering something. In a 1520 engraving after Raphael, Marc Antonio Raimondi's *The Judgement of Paris* (from which Manet borrows), the reclining figure of the man in front offers a forestal fern. Through these various citations crossing through Roddick's photograph, the central line of vision onto Roddick herself can be read as an incitement, a promiscuous mobility, the desire to trade.

Interestingly, the Kaiapó desire for white women is represented as a token moment in the question of assimilation. Basically, the logic goes, Indians who are real Indians do not desire white women, whereas those who are not real Indians do. The defense, reports the *Washington Post*, claims that Paiakan's status as a nonassimilated Indian makes him incapable of the desire that would have compelled him to commit the alleged crime:

> [Carlos Amaury] Azevedo ... will argue that Paiakan's "lack of full integration" made it unlikely he could have committed the rape. "He feels inhibited and inferior in the presence of a white woman. It is very difficult for him to experience erotic feelings and possess a white woman," the lawyer said.

"Certainly," Brazilian anthropologist Darcy Ribeiro told *Veja*, "this rape is contaminated by the whites. Indians are not neurotic, nor do they have problems with sex" (73). "The lack of discernment over the universe of the whites or mental retardation" (*Veja*, 71) was a legal category to designate nonassimilation, a limit-case of mental sanity defining ethnic identity, proven in a medical examination. Paiakan was actually subject to such a medical examination to see whether he was insane enough to have committed the rape and ritual torture: "In the case of Paiakan, an investigation of this type could determine if he knew that he was committing crimes when he tortured and raped Letícia" (*Veja*, 71).

However, the description of Paiakan as incapable of interracial desire is distinctly opposed to the Paiakan who, earlier in the *Washington Post* article, is outside the forest, participating in urban rituals, Brazilian culture, consumer consumption, and their inescapable corollary—the desire for white women: "As his income grew, Paiakan moved to Redencao[,] ... bought two cars and a house in Belem, a distant Amazon capital. He frequented Redencao bars, danced in the annual carnival and was often seen with local girls."

Indian desire for the white woman is proof that assimilation leads to the disappearance of Kaiapó culture as it is replaced by a consumption out of control and by practices of accumulation:

> "Let's suppose that I am white," [Paiakan] said. "Let's suppose that you are my wife. You are jealous, and you don't want me to look [at other women]. When I do, you say, 'Why do you look?' That's the white way. With us, we can look at everybody. But at the moment the wife realizes something is going on, there is no conversation. She doesn't say anything, she's just ... off to war!" said Paiakan. (Buchanan, 214)[27]

Paiakan's roving eye, his cinematographic eye, his hungry and hunting look demonstrates the capital excess—the desire for accumulation and assimilation, the desire for whiteness—that threatens Kaiapó reproduction. Irekran, in revenge, makes visible the marking of territory, the defense of the family, and cultural difference.

In *Identification Papers,* Diana Fuss has demonstrated how identification or assimilation paradoxically merges into stories of cannibalistic practice within imperial discourse. Identification, as a conceptual space where desire and identity are interpenetrative, becomes the narrative of a primitive desire to usurp—by eating—the Other in the totemic meal.[28] Writes Sam Dillon in the *Miami Herald*:

> Some Brazilian journalists have interpreted [the events of the rape] as a bizarre resurgence of an ancient tribal fertility rite. . . .
>
> At some point, Paiakan climbed into the back seat with Ferreira, removing his shorts. He was acting, he claimed to police, on Irekran's orders.
>
> According to Ferreira, Paiakan then raped her, and the two Indians tormented her and licked her blood. (14A)[29]

Paiakan undresses capitalism, revealing in full its predatory, rapacious nature. The sordid feast of the global consumer appears as raw power, cannibalistic, destroying people and forests as it digests them into the system. What becomes clear is that the Paiakan case is not simply a matter of cultural recognition or benevolent "partnerships" established in the name of preservation, sustainability, and cultural survival. Rather, fully assimilated, Kaiapó culture has revealed itself as thoroughly expressive of capitalist values in their most natural forms, promising, as Thomas Friedman says of globalization, "more choices as to what to eat" (286). As capitalist values, in their global media coverage, are made to seem natural through their association with the Kaiapó, the possibility becomes ever more tenuous that human relationships might be based on something other than violence, savagery, racism, exploitation, and hard competition over seemingly scarce resources.

There is no doubt that alternative media have been a powerful, effective, and successful tool not only for indigenous and environmental activism all over the world but also for a host of other oppositional practices. As Beth Conklin has pointed out in reference to indigenous media,

> Identity politics—especially its ecological variants—have brought unprecedented visibility and transnational support to native peoples' struggles for land and legal rights critical to their survival. In many ways the participation of Amazonian Indians in transnational ecopolitics represents a radical departure from dependency relations of the past. The Indian-environmentalist alliance articulates a model of partnership, not paternalism, and champions indigenous self-determination—the right of native peoples to make choices about their own destinies. (714)

However, the Paiakan case makes clear that indigenous peoples' entrance into alliances with Western technologies and capital do not guarantee justice and equal partnership. The Kaiapó have here reconstructed their own ethnic identities (their own differences) as effects of power, as a celebration of neoliberal expansiveness—the universalization of consumer choices as markets spread, a proof of capital's compassion in providing conditions of survival for all. In fact, such alliances often testify to the intransigence of capital's powers of assimilation and accommodation to difference, its very plasticity. Underlying this message, the Paiakan case exhibits the way global capitalism subordinates cultural differences to commercialism and spectacle and expresses cultural differences only as a type of exotic violence that needs taming and rationalization, an excuse for interventions that benefit increased exploitation and further restrictions on indigenous economic practices. Writes Alexander Cockburn:

> No sooner had the last environmentalist quit Eco '92 in Rio than, on July 15, the Secretary General of the Presidency, Marcos Coimbra, issued Aviso 745, which changed the procedures for demarcation of indigenous land, making them subject to the approval of the military, the department of mines, the agricultural ministry and the national electrical power company.... Aviso 745 essentially opens up indigenous lands to any predatory economic group. (329)

As the image of the global consumer lies at the center of how this story gets told, the case shores up an ideological conviction for a consumerist politics invading even the most marginal corners of the globe. One wonders, indeed, what kinds of new exclusions are produced in capitalism's recognition of the Kaiapó as its exemplary success story, as its trophy, its triumph, and its redemption. What kinds of peoples, for example, might not be so appealing to a politics of recognition based on the visibility of difference as exoticism and an accommodation to the forces and desires of the market?

Conclusion

It is not surprising today to say that the family is a problem. It's what my students tell me, what I read in the newspapers, what the politicians say, and what I see at the movies. A recent movie like *8MM* drives the point home, so to speak, although many current mainstream as well as art films seem to repeat the same message. The main character's (Nicholas Cage) forays into the underground worlds and sordid cultures of snuff film production end up provoking the bloodthirsty pornographers into a counterattack against his family. Worried, he incessantly calls his wife, even in the midst of crime and battle, to inquire about the welfare of their baby, Cinderella. Time and again, the wife responds with, "Cindy's fine and she loves you," an exchange that seems to make even the grossest acts of Cage's revenge both appealing and justified, because he is defending such a sweet and loving baby. The more the main character approaches the ambit of the perverts, the more his beautiful white baby girl, his house with its nice lawn, and his wife's adoration are endangered. We are living at a time, the film is telling us, when evil forces are out to take over our identities and then get our children; and we'd better beware, take precautions, kill a lot of people in the process of protection.

What exactly are these evil forces? What is inciting such excessive measures of defense? There are a number of possible explanations, my students tell me. One is, of course, bad parenting, and bad parenting results from working mothers. Because the economy is so difficult, the argument goes, because people aren't making enough to live. Because jobs are unstable, mothers are forced to enter the work force. When mothers work, children are undisciplined; they are not properly taught good values and moral behavior. The recent movie *Step Mom* illustrates this point well. When the parents get divorced, the stepmother (Julia Roberts) tries to take over the role of the real mother (Susan Sarandon), but she is awkward and neglectful of the needs of the kids, mostly because she is much too ambitious, too focused on her own career of fashion photography. Not only do the kids subsequently get lost when she is on a shoot but the cute little white kids are also exposed to sexuality and, in particular, illicit female sexuality. Because of the lack of surveillance and structure, the little girl walks into the bathroom when the father and the stepmother are at it in the shower, causing a host of possible traumatic repercussions for the child (though the movie never specifies quite what they are; instead, we are meant to assume that such an incident is inherently adverse to the child's healthy development and especially her moral development).

These attitudes certainly extend beyond the cinema. The recent tragedy at Columbine High School in Littleton, Colorado, where two white students in black trenchcoats shot up a high school, killing twelve other students and a teacher before turning their guns on themselves, is also the fault, my students and the media tell me, of poor parenting. If the kids were building bombs in the garage and stockpiling semi-automatic weapons in their bedrooms, why didn't the parents know about it? It is the absence of proper mothering, a loosening of everyday surveillance, that leads to what everybody recognizes as the natural and explainable cruelty of children. I then asked my students if they thought that social security would be available to them when they got older, if they thought they would be guaranteed health care coverage with their work—if they thought, in short, they would be doing better than their parents. They all said no but denied that any of these political/economic changes in their world affected the behavior of children in high school, who were only concerned with their own social lives. Adolescents, they insisted, were naturally egocentric. It's the way they're brought up. This is the case always and everywhere. Their psychology textbooks said so.

The prevalent belief in a mothering crisis tends to mask how it is really economics, and particularly the economics of the new globalisms, that are causing such untold damage to the family. Who, after all, I asked my students, who is giving the example, promoting a militarization of culture, building bombs and dropping them? In Kosovo, again, the media seems to suggest, there is a crisis of poor parenting, where unruly, cruel, infant-like evildoers—like the Littleton killers, depicted through Nazi imagery—are killing one another. What needs to be done is for the moral, humanitarian, and imperialist father to step in and impose discipline, take away the toys and guns that are causing so much death, destruction, and misery. The militarization of masculinity and the demonization of mothering are flipsides of the same coin, as the absence of the mother's watchful eye demands the imposition of police rule both in the domestic and the international spheres. The absence of the mother—with her moral methods of socialization, her reproduction of good through teaching and example—leads to the forceful intervention of the father who will, it is clear, create an iron rule of law. This global father will, on the one hand, put metal detectors and other systems of surveillance in both inner-city and suburban schools (but more often in the former) and, on the other hand, deploy NATO troops with their tools of surveillance and discipline in Yugoslavia, for the purpose of European stability and the expansion of U.S. influence abroad. The state is here operating in the interests of multinational corporate control, as companies like Boeing, General Dynamics, and Lockheed-Martin are the ones profiting from the U.S. purchases and development of new military technologies and more guns, even while professing, on the domestic front, the need for more gun control. The so-called "two regional conflicts" theory bodes well for private industry. As NATO continues to define its slaughtering of ethnic Albanians as "collateral damage," it is clear that the very forces destroying the family—the violent forces of capital itself—are depicted as the forces that will save it and rescue all those innocent women and children from being raped and massacred in the Greater Serbia.

A massive cultural campaign is going on that demands the family's defense at the same time as the family itself is under assault by the forces of capital and is being made indefensible under their monstrous and momentous transformative powers. Although the U.S. movie industry seems to recognize the current weakness of the family and its organization of the social, that industry seems to be attributing the family's demise to the presence of perversity opposing it and seeking its end, erasing the role of capital in this process. The destructiveness of capital is being blamed on bad mothering. Bad mothering is seen as caused by intrusions into conceptions of identity, of difference; difference itself is defined as both psychopathological and perverse. This logic plays on the notion developed in evolutionary science that the mother is the site where, in cross-breeding, species identity could be contaminated and then transformed, where outside forces could enter into and change the self into something different, a hybrid form and a new identity. As the conformity of species to itself was supposed to be determined, before Darwin, on the premise that hybrid forms could only reproduce sterile offspring, it is the idea of difference that reproductive motherhood should block out but also, as Darwin discovered, what it lets in. This logic has also built itself into a broader cultural imaginary—used even to support legalized divisions between the colonizer and the colonized—where the role of the mother as socializer was supposed to guard the moral values of civilization and all that implied in terms of race, class, domination, and the imposition of power.

Perversion in these mass cultural representations is seen as trying to enter the family if the mother lets down her guard, showing that motherhood is malfunctioning, not drawing the borders around a disciplined identity, but instead allowing the dangerously perverse to seep through her control. Just as new deregulations on capital mean that money can go anywhere, enter into production anywhere, reproduce itself anywhere, so motherhood is shown to be no longer in control of policing stable identities or producing legible, definitional boundaries of race, ethnicity, class, gender, nation, sexuality, and the moral life. One can no longer think of the family, as Freud and then Lacan did, as insular, nor represent the mother, as they did, as the deceptive Other who abandons the child inside the walled-in enclosure of a comfortable home, creating an initial lack. Instead, today the mother operates as a gateway that lets the dangerous and migrant Other—the very idea of fluidity, of circulation, and the impossibility of enforcing the law—into the very core of who we are, demanding ever-stricter policies of surveillance, discipline, and control in private lives.

The perspective on these issues at the international level contrasts sharply with these images from U.S.-produced popular culture. A writer like Mahasweta Devi has been able to show compellingly how the family is being unraveled by the movement of capital rather than by an undefinable perversity approaching ever so dangerously close to our front doors. In the short story "The Hunt," Devi presents the colonial child Mary Oraon, half-white and half-tribal, who was conceived when a landholding colonist raped her servant mother. What made the family obsolete, in this instance, was that colonialism ended and the father went to Australia, selling the house and the forest to a man from the native merchant class, thereby initiating a capitalist appropriation of the forest. The incident is repeated when Tehsildar Singh comes into the forest with designs to corporatize the lumber trade and make partnerships with the natives whom he would later exploit. Singh's destructive presence in the jungle is shown through his insistent seductions of Mary, which threaten to obstruct her promise of marriage to Jalim, a Muslim. Singh's flirtations with Mary become more and more forceful the more she refuses him, until she kills him in a symbolic act of rape, thus reversing the relations of power, on the feast day of the ritual hunt.

The story explores the impact of capitalist development and market expansion on the identity of a woman who is also an economic agent, a member of a community, and a sexual—perhaps reproductive—being. Mary's ability to sell the fruit she picks from the trees, at least quasi-legally, at the local market is seriously infringed by the reorganization of production that the new capitalist infrastructure is maneuvering, just as her promise to marry her intended Jalim—a promise that depended on her accumulation of a certain amount of surplus earnings from fruit sales—is deflected. In her short story "Douloti, The Bountiful," Devi is able to show even more poignantly the relationship between a postcolonial capitalist culture and a female sexuality defined through it. Douloti is the daughter of a bond slave who is tortured for accumulating capital outside of the debt contract. Unable to meet any more payments through his labor because of his physical depravity, he exchanges his daughter for cash with a Brahmin who turns out not to want to marry her but instead to keep her as a whore. Drawing female sexuality into a culture of debt and then into an impetus to profit, capitalism is here clearly shown as destructive to family relations. In the end, Douloti tries to return to her home and her family, but infected with weakness and disease, she dies on the road, in a schoolyard, on top of a chalk-etching map of the nation India.

Perversity here is not somehow an aberrant cultural form that capitalism will redeem and protect us from. Neither Mary's masculinized revenge nor Douloti's whoring is a consequence of poor mothering. Instead, perversity is a result of the family's very intense relations with the globalizing forces of capitalism. Capitalism makes the family perverse and, hence, the need to extricate it, to bound it on the outside, to label it as "aberrant," "sick," and so forth. Perhaps the current stigmatization, in the United States, of alternative sexualities camouflages a critique of capital of the kind that Devi does, hiding the interactions between sex and money that are at the heart of everybody's practices and the ways people live. And perhaps, too, the idea that the family is only sanctified in its expulsion of capital as dirty and perverse makes the immigrant into a perverse figure in the U.S. imaginary, with the immigrant functioning as a reminder that capital creates dispersements which disrupt the familial, setting it, like the commodity, into circulation, turning it into something other than the secure enclave protecting civilization and its values. With the vast movements of people created in global capital shifts, the family becomes a fetish, its disappearance recognized and disavowed. As the immigrant makes visible the processes of production, she also exemplifies the idea that the family is in need of protection because it is losing its viability, increasingly posed in the horrors of the imaginary as needing ever more fierce strategies of security to ensure its ideal of reproducing itself. It is this connection that is hidden—a relation between the production of life (both discursive and reproductive) and global production.

Notes

Introduction

1. "The movements of deconstruction do not destroy structures from the outside. They are not possible and effective, nor can they take accurate aim, except by inhabiting those structures. Inhabiting them *in a certain way*, because one always inhabits, and all the more when one does not suspect it. Operating necessarily from the inside, borrowing all the strategic and economic resources of subversion from the old structure, borrowing them structurally, that is to say without being able to isolate their elements and atoms, the enterprise of deconstruction always in a certain way falls prey to its own work" (Derrida, 1976: 24).

2. I am referring here to Diana Fuss's book with this title, where she argues, "The binary articulation of essentialism and difference can ... be restrictive, even obfuscating, in that it allows us to ignore or to deny the differences *within* essentialism.... [C]onstructivism ... really operates as a more sophisticated form of essentialism. The bar between essentialism and constructivism is by no means as solid and unassailable as advocates of both sides assume it to be" (1989: xii).

Darwin's Dating Game

1. There has recently been some scholarly interest in exploring the boundaries between science and literature. See, for example, Beer (1983), who examines the ways Eliot and Hardy adopted narrative structures and literary devices from Darwin; Levine, who analyzes the detachment of Victorian narrative structures as related to Victorian protocols of scientific observation; Krasner, who specifically focuses on novelistic point of view as evolving out of the study of optics and visual psychology, with a contingent scientific attention to witnessing and documenting natural diversity; and Lightman,

who is interested in social context, particularly in relation to the influences of popular culture and scientific practices.

2. Ornella Moscucci argues that the project of searching for a biological foundation to sexual difference was caught up in the Enlightenment concern with the "science of man." Sexual difference, according to Moscucci, was used as a sign of the limit to the properly human. "During the Victorian period," she writes, "attempts to reconcile the concept of sexual difference with the idea of human nature common to both sexes typically took the form of a widespread fascination with the latent hermaphrodism or bisexuality of humankind" (17). Also, Londa Schiebinger (1993) shows how gender and reproduction worked as a logic behind the development of taxonomies, both botanical and zoological, in the eighteenth century. She argues that Linnaeus created plant taxonomies through highlighting and describing reproductive systems, sex organs, and sex parts, and that the term "mammal" derived from social anxieties about population diminishment on account of wet-nursing, rather than from the universality of breastfeeding among the animals labeled such. Schiebinger (1986) also shows how, in the tradition of eighteenth-century anatomical illustrations, depictions of sexual difference—where women, for instance, had larger pelvises and men had larger crania—became the touchstone of the developing realism in scientific representations. Also, Cynthia Eagle Russett demonstrates how arguments about the separate spheres of labor were used as metaphors for the growing complexities of the more evolved organism. The division of labor between different cells and tissues came to be the model for the sexual division of labor in "advanced" biological societies, separating the ideal of domestic Victorian motherhood from the barbarous treatment given to "savage women," who were made to perform the drudge work and physical labor more appropriate to the male sphere (131).

3. Theories of population ecology say that if a resource is limited, a population decrease could result. This process could lead to evolution but does not necessarily always operate in conjunction with natural selection. A migration of a nearby population, for example, could counter the evolutionary process by bringing genes back into the initial community.

4. Indeed, at the same time as evolution emerges as the dominant paradigm of the biological sciences, population, as Foucault has pointed out, was becoming a focus for framing power and rationalizing the economy, categorizing people and identities for the purposes of managing normalcy. "One of the great innovations in the techniques of power in the eighteenth century," Foucault starts his discussions of "biopopulation," "was the emergence of 'population' as an economic and political problem: population as wealth, population as manpower or labor capacity, population balanced between its own growth and the resources it commanded" (25).

5. Joel Kovel has used such scenarios to explain the uncertainty figured into narratives of scientific positivism. The anxious speculation going on now in many places—that environmental crisis is causing widespread troubles in male fertility count and population sustainability—is couched, Kovel observes, in subjunctive tenses and provisional qualifiers. "Let us begin with a fact or, at any rate, a finding," Kovel says. "It has been found, by 'science,' that for about thirty to fifty years, sperm counts have been

declining, in both numbers and motility, among men in industrialized countries" (192). "There can be no Holy Grail of scientific certainty in questions of this sort," Kovel concludes after reading the evidence.

6. Current feminist historians in medicine and biology are working on exposing the nineteenth-century backlash against feminism that the social anxiety over birth rates fostered. Carroll Smith-Rosenberg and Charles Rosenberg have addressed the influence of feminism on family limitation and the birth control movement: "Though birth control and abortion had been practiced, discussed—and reprobated—for centuries," they note, "the mid-nineteenth century saw a dramatic increase in concern among spokesmen for the ministry and medical profession" (343). Schiebinger talks about how women's search for political rights of citizenship, after the Revolution in France, created such a scientific backlash, which regulated women as reproductive creatures (172–83).

7. The story goes that the paper was forgotten until 1900, when three different scientists "rediscovered" it simultaneously, and so was born modern genetics. Mendel, however, was concerned with outward traits rather than inward transmissions and with essential stability rather than transformation.

8. In 1865, Darwin advanced a theory of trait inheritance called "pangenesis," postulating that organic tissues would produce an excess of hard germ particles, or "gemmules," which would be released in the germ plasm. The germ plasm would then transport these particles, each containing an exact quality of the part of the body from which it was formed, to the sexual cells, from where they would be combined and transmitted (*Variation,* 349–50).

9. Also, for discussions on Darwin's influences on Freud, see Lucille Ritvo (1965, 1972), who shows how Freud is indebted to Darwin for his theories on Lamarckian inheritance of acquired characteristics, where experience and ancestral memory can be passed down to future generations, and also Gould (1977: 155–64), who discusses Freud's use of the idea, current in biology, that "ontogeny recapitulates phylogeny."

10. For Ellis, both female homosexuality and inversion are for the most part degenerative. "Among moor-hens and great-crested grebes," he notes, "sometimes what Selous terms 'functional hermaphroditism' occurs and the females play the part of the male toward their male companions, and then repeat the sexual act with a reversion to the normal order, the whole to the satisfaction of both parties" (233). By the second volume of his studies, Ellis is examining inversion as a permanent condition—affecting even object choice—among the primitive races, criminals, prostitutes, neurotics, and women in harems. Jane Caplan discusses Ellis's and Krafft-Ebing's reliance on degeneracy models to produce homosexuality as a concept. Also, Jennifer Terry talks about how such a model, in Ellis's work, allows two different interpretations: (1) homosexuality as an adaptive regression due to nervous stress, leading to a primitive freedom of unleashed sexual appetite; and (2) as overspecialization, where too much energy has been used up in civilization's demands, leaving none for reproduction and leading to sterility (132). Siobhan Somerville has analyzed the conjunction of homosexuality and race in sexological studies. "Is it merely a coincidence," she asks, "that the classification of bodies as either 'homosexual' or 'heterosexual' emerged at the same time that the United States was aggressively policing the imaginary boundaries between 'black' and 'white' bodies?"

(245) In particular, she cites Ellis as using naturalist paradigms and metaphors of ancestry to explain inversion as a racial question.

11. Jane Gallop, for example, comments on how psychoanalysis is based on the closed circuit of the family unit and that what gets omitted from such schema is that the home itself is a formulation of class and has class divisions within it: "Class conflict and revolution are understood as a repetition of parent-child relations" (144). For Gallop, the servant class within the home—particularly the nurses and maids, are exchanged like the mother, representing the notion of an alterity that is already within the structure, an alterity that brings into play money circulation—which "would constitute the greatest threat to the law homogenizing the family" (145) and open up the psychoanalytic paradigm to the class conflict at the heart of it.

12. I owe thanks to Ken Saltman for helping me work out the ideas in this section.

13. In their current form these policies have served as excuses to blame public schooling for a host of social problems, including drug use and a perceived increase in crime rates, delinquency, unemployment, and the like. They have also served as justification to close public schools in the inner cities, to move teachers around, and to withdraw funds from public schools whose performance rates are low, further imbalancing equalities of opportunity and the rights of all Americans to a decent education. I am aware that national testing and standards have not necessarily been a beneficial and just solution to the problems of localized educational policy in terms of ending racial oppressions and unfair distributions of money and power.

14. I thank Henry Giroux for pointing out this article.

Conrad's Closet

1. Much lesbian theory has noted the relationship or even the collapse in nineteenth-century degeneracy theories between sexual aberrations or perversions and the evolutionary arrests that came to represent nonwhite racial identities. "By the end of the nineteenth century," writes, for example, Judith Raiskin, "the metaphor of racial degeneration had became conflated with that of sexual degeneracy, perhaps because of the illicit sexuality exposed by 'mixed-race' offspring or because of European fascination with the sexual physiology and imagined sexual practices of Africans" (157). Similarly, Marylynne Diggs remarks, "Representing confusions of the binary paradigm of gender and race identification, the human sciences of the nineteenth century simply normalized certain identities and produced vast taxonomies for categorizing as pathological those who did not fit the norm" (4). In this chapter, however, I contend that race and gender do not simply collapse into a vast degenerate category in which all deviations are scientifically interchangeable. They do, of course, operate through cross-referencing one another, complexly intersecting, fragmenting, interacting with, *and* contradicting one another within the fields of power where they are each generated.

2. Reading this material through a Foucauldian paradigm, David Horn has argued that Lombroso's "criminal anthropology" marks the "normal" woman as a site where the emerging realm of the "social" would inscribe its discourses of risk and endangerment. He observes that Lombroso's "normal" woman is already threatened because femininity is a sign of less advanced stages in the progress of evolution. For Horn, criminal

anthropology collapses the categories of identity, which it would seem to uphold, by showing that the presence of the Other is always internal. The "female offender," Horn argues, was a legible, bodily sign of the "violent, bloodthirsty" "natural instincts" of "prehistoric man" (112) already existing as potential within the parameters defining normalcy in women.

3. For a 1929 follow-up study to this one, which comes to very similar conclusions, see Ford.

4. Nancy Armstrong has demonstrated how conduct books for women became popular in conjunction with the rise of the printing press and the subsequent birth of mass culture in the mid-nineteenth century, providing a frame of reference for the development of the novel (896–97).

5. For a study on how national and racial borders were drawn and redrawn through European women's sexual moralities and the impossible project of protecting, defending, and rescuing their purities, see Guy.

6. For an interesting study on the intersections of colonial realist photography and Victorian pornography, see Barkan.

7. Recent criticism has noted Conrad's debt to Haggard, especially in borrowing his conceptions of the feminization of colonial space and the adventurism at the center of colonial discourses of masculinity. See, for example, McClintock, 1–4; Showalter, 83–98; Gilbert (1983); and Gilbert and Gubar, 10–46.

8. The Victorian governess has been coming up in theory as a representative of how the social forces of femininity intersect with those of race and class. Jane Gallop, for example, speculates, "The family never was, in any of Freud's texts, completely closed off from questions of economic class. And the most insistent locus of that intrusion into the family circuit (intrusion of the symbolic into the imaginary) is the maid/governess/nurse. As Cixous says, 'she is the hole in the social cell.' . . . The servant, member of the lower class, like a child, is capable of perversion" (144–45). Jim Swann has discussed how Freud's own governess, his "teacher in sexual matters," was central to his projections of a humiliating father in the Oedipal complex. In the analysis that follows, I refer mainly to Mary Poovey's, Katheryn Hughes's, Anne McClintock's, and Ann Laura Stoler's social histories of female domestic service and hired child care, the later two for their readings of governesses within a colonial symbolics; see also Renton, Clarke, and Gathorne-Hardy.

9. The entire story of *Chance* is predicated on the assumption of a false family name. Powell gets the job on the *Ferndale* because he has the same family name as the person in charge of company hiring. Powell uneasily claims parentage where most likely none exists.

10. In Freud, narcissism is a remainder from a primordial time before the separation between the ego instincts of self-preservation and the sexual instincts of reproduction. It is particularly pervasive in children and animals who, under its influence, become more attractive because of their resulting sexual self-sufficiency and inaccessibility (70). In Lacanian psychoanalysis and later in deconstruction, the narcissistic projection becomes the misrecognized object, the sign of difference. Deconstruction's erasure of the possibility of specularity is, actually, reflected within Homi Bhabha's ideas about colonial mimesis.

Carpentier's Marvelous Conception

1. Throughout this and the following chapters, translations from Spanish-language works are mine.

2. The Sartrean influence on Carpentier's concept of alienation, on the depiction of Mouche's circle of friends, and on the idea, worked throughout the novel, of constructing an "essence" through an "act" of "existence," has been explored by Ian MacDonald (1979). Mouche's name is almost certainly drawn from the title of Sartre's play *Les Mouches*.

3. Eduardo González has written about the importance of contracts as a leitmotif in *The Lost Steps*. The narrator protagonist is tied to the world of a city through a series of contracts, the one with Ruth, the one with his employers at the publicity firm, and now the one with the ethnomusicological museum and the university. The contract, argues González, is a document that creates the identity of the person before the person, in an existential sense, exists. It signifies, therefore, an essence that precedes an existence, a preformed essence that the subject can only repeat, a living in bad faith. In fact, when the plane appears, the narrator-protagonist convinces himself that he needs to return to the city in order to annul this conjugal contract, an ambition that he never achieves. See Gonzáles, 596.

4. Carpentier wrote this novel while incarcerated for his involvement with student organizing against the then Cuban dictator Machado.

5. For a convincing analysis of Carpentier's early debt to the discourse of criminal anthropology, see González Echevárria (1977), 66–68.

6. For an analysis of the history of surrealist influence on Carpentier's "lo real maravilloso americano," see Müller-Bergh. For an analysis of Carpentier's adoption of surrealism's "the marvelous" to naturalize the "revelation of Latin American difference," see Chiampi. For an analysis of how Carpentier's aesthetic theory fits the surrealist proposition of a magical elsewhere, one beyond the bourgeois-rational world, and of how surrealism's rupture with Bréton is reflected in Carpentier's rupture with European tradition, see Bravo, 19–27.

7. Zamora goes on to explain that the baroque is a particularly adequate method for representing revolutionary histories.

8. Carmen Perilli adds that "the infantile scene of the canoe in the river is the recreation of the infantile scene of María del Carmen in the cradle" (170; my translation). María del Carmen is the narrator's childhood sweetheart with whom he "plays house," pretending to be married. Writes Carpentier, "I now asked María del Carmen if she wanted to be my wife, and as she answered yes, I squeezed her a little tighter, imitating the sound of a ship's siren so she would not go away from me, I found it hard to breathe, my heart throbbed, and yet this discomfort was so agreeable" (93).

9. See, for example, González Echevarría (1977), 165, and Giovannini, 70.

10. Carpentier would later, however, work in the Ministry of Culture under Castro. He was, until he died, a faithful defender of Castro's revolution, even though he was in exile during the insurgency.

11. One of the obvious difficulties in discussing this text here is the authors' insistence on the anglophone orientation of postcolonial literatures. The other is that the

histories of anticolonial struggles in Latin America did not follow the same historical trajectories by which the authors define postcolonial movements or postcolonial nations.

12. For an interesting discussion on how primitive male sexuality becomes the site of universal masculinity, in the early twentieth century United States, through the figure of the "natural man," see Bederman. The Amazon has often represented an imaginary site for a universal, unrestricted male sexuality. For instance, Eustasio Rivera's *La vorágine,* one of Carpentier's sources in writing *The Lost Steps,* is a story of one narrator's search for a woman who has disappeared in the Colombian jungle, a search that is littered with allusions to his potency in the symbolic chaos of the precolonized primitive: "Cual se agota una esperma invertida sobre su llama, acabó presto con mi ardentía esta loba insaciable, que oxida con su aliento mi virilidad" (223). A novel like Vargas Llosa's *Pantaleón y las visitadoras* (1973) will pick up and develop this connection between the Amazon and male sexuality as comedy. For some anthropological explorations of this theme, see, for example, Bamberger, McCallum (1994), Gregor, Good, and Schneebaum.

Mario Vargas Llosa and the Rape of Sebastiana

1. The subjective pronouns are omitted in the Spanish here. In my translation here I have kept the objective pronouns in the feminine, as they are when *la realidad* is their antecedent. The English impersonal or neuter pronouns, usually used for things or ideas, do not sufficiently address the way gender would work in the Spanish.

2. For a fascinating discussion of how genius gets signified as an autonomous, self-generating man in nineteenth-century Britain, see "The Man-of-Letters Hero: *David Copperfield* and the Professional Writer" in Poovey.

3. The artist is condemned to his material, as his material selects him (94), but the working-through, the choice of form, is what makes *libertad* an existential act. The Sartrean influence is less important to my argument than the use of Bataille.

4. Brennan's literalization of the metaphor of Canudos as a reference to *Sendero Luminoso* is most likely historically inaccurate here: "It is very unlikely that the, on some level admirable, fanaticism of the *jagunços* with its horrible consequences was not inspired very directly by Vargas Llosa's own reading of Peru's Mao rebels, *Sendero Luminoso* ('Shining Path')" (66). However, in 1980, only a year before *La guerra del fin del mundo* was first published and when Peru was returning to civilian rule after twelve years of military dictatorship, *Sendero,* at first a student movement challenging the imposing of tuition on secondary education, performed its first public acts of violence when they seized the ballot box for a national election in the village of Chuschi, Huamanga province. According to David Scott Palmer, "The Belaúnde administration did not take the increasingly violent group seriously for almost three full years. Only then did the government declare the Ayacucho area an emergency zone and send in the military" (14). Contrary to Brennan's claim, it is *highly* unlikely, then, that *Sendero* would have reached, by 1981, a type of global exposure that would justify Vargas Llosa's writing a 600-page novel referencing the *Sendero* movement, nor that he would have been alarmed enough at that point to do so.

5. In another article, "Apuntes sobre la crítica feminista y la literatura hispanoamericana," Franco warns against sliding a consideration of the oppression of women

too easily, as Kristeva as well as Retamar would do, into a more generalized discussion of oppression, specifically of colonial and racial oppression (34–35).

6. "The picture of violence which we must attribute to primitive man in particular must necessarily be understood as opposed to the rhythm of work regulated by rational factors" (*Bataille,* 44).

7. For a discussion of how a discourse on civilization deployed racial and gender categories, recreating masculinity in terms of evolutionary racial progress in a Euroamerican context at and around the turn of the century, see Bederman.

8. Brazil was the last country in the Americas to abolish slavery in 1889. The republic was formed in 1890.

9. There is a consensus among critics that the myopic journalist is supposed to represent Euclides da Cunha, whose first-hand reporting on the episode, published in 1902, is titled in English *Rebellion in the Backlands,* trans. Samuel Butnam (Chicago: University of Chicago Press, 1944). In *La guerra del fin del mundo,* Vargas Llosa is essentially rereading this original text.

10. Some critics have read *La guerra del fin del mundo* as a displaced vituperation against liberation theology, with Canudos representing a Christian base community. See, for example, Brennan, 66.

11. Gall is referring, particularly, to Jurema in this question.

12. For instance, the vow of chastity also links both Galileo Gall and the Baroness to el Consejero, who is also abstinent.

13. See her analysis of *Conversación,* (1981).

14. This is not to say that women weren't involved in "Libertad." Some women contributed significantly to Vargas Llosa's efforts in this regard and also subsequently entered political life; his wife, Patricia, played a fundamental role. See the *Mesa Redonda,* where Nella de Castro, Lourdes Flores, and Beatriz Merino talk about women's participation in Peruvian politics in general and their activism within Vargas Llosa's "Libertad" party in particular; see also Villar Márquez.

15. No mention was given as to how this would happen.

16. See Blondet (1991), Blondet (1991), and Stokes.

17. Again, people in Peru either didn't remember this program or said that it had always been a function of government and therefore was not particular to Vargas Llosa's agenda.

18. These memoirs are actually structured on the principle of a strict separation of the public from the private. Chapters telling about the campaign are alternated with subjective autobiographical chapters telling of his youth in Lima and the growth of his literary career.

19. The title is quite obviously supposed to mean that the economic revolution exhibited in the text would be a positive alternative to the revolution that was simultaneously being carried out by *Sendero Luminoso,* and which had been, since 1980, severely weakening Peru's economy through violence, terror, and civil war.

20. As Degregori notes, in Vargas Llosa's presidential initiative, "one of the recurrent motives is the struggles against a state of 'the life of barbarism, of the African society'; where the objective of Fredemo is sketched as that of 'saving our nation from barbarism'" (73).

The Rainforest Rape

1. In a conversation I had early in 1994 with Brian Ferguson, an anthropologist at Rutgers University working on Amazonian issues, he informed me that at a South American Indian conference held at Bennington College in August 1992, two Brazilian women spoke on the case of Paiakan. According to Ferguson, the women were baffled by the events. They had said that in Brazil, it was extremely rare for Indians to rape white women but that at the time when the allegations against Paiakan became public, there seemed to be a proliferation of such cases reported all over the country. Daniela Peluso, an anthropologist also working in the Amazon and an attendee at the conference, has corroborated Ferguson's account. The increase in publicized stories about Indians raping white women occurred at a time of increased racial tensions owing to federal reorganization and intense legal debates over racial status. The battles being waged at high government levels seem to have translated into a paranoia in everyday relations. The anthropologist Cecelia McCallum reports that after the *Veja* coverage, people frequently asked her during her fieldwork with the Indians in Bahía if she was afraid of being raped (5). The situation seems to me to correspond with Jenny Sharpe's compelling analysis about the frequent allegations of natives' raping of white women after the 1857 Sepoy rebellion in India and the resultant reign of fear. She argues that "a crisis in British authority is managed through the circulation of the violated bodies of English women as a sign for the violation of colonialism. In doing so, I see English womanhood emerge as an important cultural signifier for articulating a colonial hierarchy of race" (4). The crisis in Brazilian federalism and the concern in Brazil over the new imperialism and the foreign interventions of the environmental movement, seem to me to suggest parallels. For an analysis of how women's sexualities have been produced and defined in the Brazilian popular press's coverage of spectacular rapes, see Pereira Coelho.

2. In an e-mail interview on 24 August 1996, with Daryl Posey, an ethnobotanist working with the Kaiapó and a co-activist with Paiakan, he wrote that "Paiakan was a very inconvenient indian to the government . . . you must know the Xingu dam scandal. He and other leaders were systematically set up so as to 'teach them a lesson.' The details of the case did not reflect Kayapo custom (rape of someone in front of their children)—and it all happened too quickly (rape one day, major full spread in *VEJA* the next—just for ECO '92). Then governor of the state wanted lands of the Kayapo—and many still do. Undermining the legitimacy of leaders and, thereby, credibility of the indians, helps to reduce the political support for indigenous land demarcation. It is a VERY OLD strategy in Brazil."

3. According to Cecelia McCallum, "*Veja* is the most widely read weekly news magazine in Brazil, in format similar to *Time*" (4).

4. Alexander Cockburn comments, "Ferreira's uncle had been *Veja*'s chief source. This uncle, Pedro Martinez Barros, with whom Ferreira became closeted after the alleged rape, is running for the post of Mayor of Redenção on an explicitly anti-Indian platform. He enlisted the services of Manoel Franco, the legal assistant to the governor of the state of Pará, a notoriously tough customer who was already engineering a campaign to reduce Kayapó land holdings."

5. Again, according to Cockburn, "The couple to whose house Ferreira made her way immediately after the incident say she was without the mutilations described in *Veja.* Scott Wallace, the U.S. freelance journalist to whom the couple made that statement, also established that there were no bloodstains in the Chevette.... The police chief, furthermore, told Wallace he had been misquoted." Scott Wallace himself says in *Penthouse,* "The car itself exhibited no signs to suggest that a bloody rape had occurred inside. I studied the crushed-velvet upholstery, looking for any clue—a small spot or some sign that would have betrayed an attempt to wash out stains. I could find nothing. I was struck by the confined space in the car, particularly in the backseat. I couldn't imagine two *consenting* adults getting it on there, let alone a two-on-one struggle of the sort described by Ferreira" (104). Wallace even questions whether Barbosa saw the car at all after the incident.

6. Beth Conklin and Laura Graham conclude, "In 1992, the Kayapó leader Payakan experienced ... a fall from grace when the Brazilian media launched a character defamation campaign against him at the outset of the United Nations Earth Summit conference (UNCED) in Rio de Janeiro. Payakan was to be the star attraction, focusing media attention on indigenous peoples' alternative summit and separate agenda. In a story that splashed across headlines around the globe, a Brazilian woman accused Payakan of violent rape.... The impact of the negative reporting ... is unmistakable. Overnight, Payakan came to be perceived as a liability to international groups with whom he was associated, and he was dropped from the boards of NGOs worldwide. Regardless of the truth behind the allegations, his career as a celebrated advocate of indigenous rights was severely damaged" (704). This proved only true in the short run.

7. During the course of doing research for this piece, I have spoken about the work with many people—Brazilians, North Americans, and British, as well as anthropologists, activists, environmentalists, and filmmakers. Most of these people have assumed that what I have been investigating is what really happened on that day in that car, and when I'm not quick to assert my own take on what the truth is, most of these people have tried to convince me that Paiakan was indeed framed by multinational interests or media correspondents, government or anti-environmentalist capitalists, or any combination of these "evil powers." In recent responses, I have even been told that Ferreira was arrested for her involvement in a car ring, and so she is obviously "low life." Whether or not she is "low life" has nothing to do with the incident of rape. To dismiss the charges and claim Paiakan's innocence is just as sexist, in my reading, as claims of Paiakan's guilt are racist. Here, I would rather look at how different powers and identities are constructed within the telling of the rape and what sorts of narratives and ideologies emerge.

8. The anthropologists Beth Conklin and Laura Graham observe, "The alliance with Amazonian Indian causes conferred another important ideological and political benefit (to the environmental movement): it legitimized first-world environmentalists' involvement in distant nations' internal affairs" (697). Conklin and Graham are writing about the alliances formed between Western causes and native movements, where both parties can achieve their goals. They call this partnership the construction of a "middle ground."

9. Elizabeth Allen notes, "In December 1967 the SPI [Indian Protection Service]

was replaced by the National Indian Foundation, FUNAI. The 1969 Brazilian Constitution recognized that Indians held usufruct rights to land, which would be owned by the state. The 1973 Indian Statute reaffirmed this: it gave the state rights to sub-surface resources on Indian lands and empowered and commanded FUNAI to legalize land titles by investigation, delimitation, and demarcation, before the granting of a presidential decree. The Indian Statute also gave FUNAI powers forcibly to relocate Indians and to exercise control over resources on indigenous lands, including leasing the land to non-Indians. To compound the issue, two decrees were passed in 1983: one altered the procedure for demarcating Indian lands, and the second allowed the state to grant mining concessions even on demarcated land.... The reaction to the assault on Indian lands and rights became part of the wider call for the end of the military regime and for a new political order" (152).

10. Allen argues that the mining interests launched a press campaign against constitutional clauses protecting the usufructuary rights of indigenous peoples on demarcated lands. The result was a draft proposal that would significantly curtail FUNAI's powers by opening up land exploration to companies with only the permission of Congress and the Indians, and not of the Union. "Other changes were also introduced," she concludes, "including two concepts which were bound to be difficult to verify or determine: that of Indian rights to 'lands of immemorial possession,' and the distinction between Indians who were or were not 'acculturated' to Brazilian society" (156).

11. Reports Julia Michaels of the *Christian Science Monitor*, "[Lidia] Luz [coordinator of the Pro-Indian Commission] says an early warning to the Indians [that new constitutional statutes would diminish their 'special recognition and rights to the land'] came when some congressmen tried unsuccessfully to write a distinction between acculturated and unacculturated Indians into the 1988 Constitution, in a bid to start bringing indigenous territory under standard Brazilian law."

12. The Kaiapó also kidnapped a group of miners and held them hostage in A-Ukre. Gordon Roddick, Anita Roddick's husband and partner in The Body Shop, went to A-Ukre and threatened to withhold contracts if such behavior continued. The case was subsequently, because of such Kaiapó opposition and displays of aggression, moved out of Redenção. The Body Shop still does business with the Kaiapó.

13. Brazil has historically had policies of population "whitening." Brazil's (genetic) improvement could be regulated, according to the philosophy of whitening, through the disappearance of the nonassimilated segments of the Brazilian population as they blended with European stock. In 1930, for example, the historian and politician João Pandiá Calogeras concluded that "the black stain is destined to disappear in a relatively short space of time because of the influx of white immigration in which the heritage of Ham is dissolving" (as cited in Skidmore, 205). Brazilian nationhood was thus described as a specifically Brazilian passion that would cross ethnic barriers, gradually turning the population white. Alongside the discourse on Brazil's increasing and strengthening whiteness, however, the ideology of degeneracy, coming out of Europe, plotted racial mixing as leading to sterility and weakness of character. Within the arguments about whitening, there therefore lingered the suggestion of racial contamination and moral collapse. Euclides da Cunha, in *Os sertõas* (*Rebellion in the Backlands,* 1902), for example, saw the confrontation of "lower" and "higher" races leading to moral

degeneration and social disintegration: "An intermingling of races highly diverse is, in the majority of cases, prejudicial. According to the conclusions of the evolutionist, even when the influence of a superior race has reacted upon the offspring, the latter shows vivid traces of the inferior one. Miscegenation carried to an extreme means regression" (84–85).

14. The Kaiapó are not the only such group to engage in the burgeoning practice of what is now called indigenous media production. For an overview of such projects, see Weatherford. For a history of visual and audio broadcasting among the Canadian Inuit, see Brisebois. David Poisey and William Hansen have made a film, *Starting Fire with Gunpowder* (1991), which documents the history and current uses of Inuit broadcasting. For an analysis of the history and practice of satellite telecommunications among the Australian aboriginals, see Ginsburg (1989–91, 1991, 1993, 1994). For a discussion of the use of television among the Yanomama of Venezuela, see Asch et al. Vincent Carelli's 1990 film *The Spirit of TV* portrays the ways the Waiapi of Brazil have used television to communicate between communities. This is to name but a few of the most prominent projects in indigenous media. A 1989 article in *Time* magazine cites a proliferation of telemedia involvement "throughout the Third World, even in the poorest and most remote areas" (80).

15. Within the theoretical literature, indigenous media and similar products of what is called the communications revolution on "the margins" are usually talked about as an effect of globalization. Such models provide a broad perspective for considering how what Mary Louise Pratt calls "autoethnographic expression" cannot be read "simply as 'authentic' self-expression or 'inauthentic' assimilation" but instead as a transcultural practice of "dialogic engagement with western modes of representation" (102) and capital movements. Faye Ginsburg, for instance, analyzes aboriginal satellite and broadcasting practices in Australia in "Indigenous Media: Faustian Contract or Global Village?": "These developments were part of a more general decentralization, democratization, and widespread penetration of media that emerged with the growth of new technologies that simultaneously worked the local and global fronts" (96). Arjun Appadurai presents five investigative frameworks—ethnoscapes, mediascapes, technoscapes, financescapes, and ideascapes—all of which, replacing "print capitalism," are fluid "landscapes." These "historically situated imaginations" involve "human movement, technological flow and financial transfers" (330) and the rapid exchange of images in the construction of fantasies and "protonarratives," historical scriptings, of "others living in other places" (331), ethnicity, and the local and the global fields. In Latin America, Nestor García Canclini has explored the conjunctions between "modernity" and "tradition" as a result "de las mezclas" (12) between market forces, technological advances and transfers, and contingent institutional transformations (see "Carpentier's Marvelous Conception," this volume). Such perspectives are often utopic. The Paiakan case shows how the introduction of video production into an indigenous community in this case did not result in a balanced global integration among balanced powers but instead revealed the inequalities that globalization can and often does sustain.

16. Fatimah Rony asserts that "while cinema makes the white woman into an image—Doane speaks of 'a certain imprecation of the cinematic image and the representation of the woman'—cinema makes the native person, man or woman, into unmediated referent" (62).

17. Turner was traveling with his wife.

18. In "Social Body and Embodied Subject," Turner invests the Kaiapó body with the real of immediacy and experience to be retrieved from postmodern generalities, theories, and abstractions: "Individual bodily changes (physical growth, the development of gender characteristics and sexual powers, mental and emotional development, etc.) correspond directly to the main articulations of social relations (the division of labor, the family cycle, gender and age grouping, etc.)" (147).

19. Monique Y. Tschofen criticizes the use of allegories of rape in fictional narratives of postcolonial subjectivities and resistances, as, for example, in Tayeb Salih's 1969 novel *Season of Migration to the North:* "The prevalence of allegorical figurations of rape within colonial and post-colonial writings demands critical attention that does not merely gloss over the multiple implications of this trope by constructing it exclusively as a figure of resistance" (502).

20. I am not implying, however, that the images of Kaiapó disappearance would in the end "feminize" Kaiapó culture. Instead, what I am suggesting is that the spatial plottings of gender in the film serve to place and define the ethnicity Kaiapó, the stereotype, within a disappearing world. The gendering of space in the film therefore places the invisible woman at the center of the visible rearrangements of land, legislative rationalizations, and the growth of Brazil's neoliberal markets stocked in the biddings for constitutional reform.

21. Will Wright agrees: "The inside/outside opposition [the opposition between civilization and wilderness] is coded at one level, . . . in most classical Westerns, through the contrast of wandering, unsettled life with domestic, established life" (50). Thomas Schatz argues that the classic Western configures "the anarchic world of Male Savagery [gets] pitted against the civilized world of Woman and Home" (51). The hero of the Western is a mediator between the wilderness and civilization, between individualism and community, and contingently between feminine domestic sedentariness and the nomadism of masculine desire. The role of the Indian in these films is, ironically, minimal. Jane Tompkins has pointed out that "the Indians I expected did not appear. The ones I saw functioned as props, bits of local color, textural effects. As people they had no existence. Quite often they filled the role of villains, predictably, driving the engine of the plot, threatening the wagon train, the stagecoach, the cavalry detachment—a particularly dangerous form of local wildlife" (8). Cawelti has, in fact, attributed the historical advent of the Indian in the Western to the Indian who "is always in the process of vanishing" (64) due to "his assimilation and extermination" at the end of the nineteenth-century Indian wars. The critical literature on the Western genre tends to explicate the Western, with its symbolic appropriation of savagery, as a defense of a failing masculinity. John Cawelti places the genre as a reaction against industrialization that created "the sense of decaying masculine potency" so evident and pervasive in American culture: "Among the most important of these developments is the tendency of industrial work to depend increasingly on the superior potency of machines, the increasing importance of women in the industrial economy, the nationalizing trend of American life which has eroded local communities and the individual's sense of control over his life and finally the decline of parental authority in the family which has undercut the basic source of masculine supremacy" (85–86). Jane Tompkins has attributed the development of the genre to a reaction against the cult of domesticity that dominated

Victorian society and the resultant first-wave feminist movement (see, for example, 37–39). For John Cawelti, "The situation must involve a hero who possesses some of the urges toward violence as well as the skills, heroism and personal honor ascribed to the wilderness way of life, and it must place this hero in a position where he becomes involved with or committed to the agents and values of civilization" (93–94). The idea that the Paiakan story was somehow involved in a recreating of these epic films was first picked up by the Brazilian editors of *Veja* when they compared the event to a John Wayne film and the film *Dances with Wolves.* The bulk of the genre's production and popularity started in the late 1930s and continued predominantly until the 1970s.

22. *The Economist* reports that "Indians have discovered not only firearms and fire-water, or *aguardiente,* but an even more powerful encouragement to self-expression: the market. Take the Kayapo, handsome warriors of the Xingu basin.... Now they have a proper reservation, and contract for their wild oils and essences with environmentally friendly companies, such as The Body Shop, a cosmetics chain" (54).

23. This is a citation from Irekran's court testimony. She is using an interpreter because she does not speak Portuguese.

24. Rob Buchanan mentions that "one of the first doctors to examine Letícia at the Redenção hospital was the same one who had, without authorization, tied off Irekran's fallopian tubes in the course of performing an abortion" (54). From Alexander Cockburn's report we learn that "the first doctor who examined Ferreira was at the time being sued by Paiakan for having, without prior consultation, tied Irekran's tubes, an operation commonly forced on Brazil's poor and Indian women (the country has the world's third-highest rate of female sterilization)."

25. One might think here of the link, which Walter Benjamin wrote about, between surgery and technologies of reproduction in modernity: "The equipment-free aspect of reality here has become the height of artifice; the sight of immediate reality has become an orchid in the land of technology.... Here the question is: How does the cameraman compare with the painter? To answer this we take recourse to an analogy with a surgical operation. The surgeon represents the polar opposite of the magician. The magician heals a sick person by the laying on of hands, the surgeon cuts into the patient's body.... Magician and surgeon compare to painter and cameraman." (233)

26. Roddick says, for example, "I think business practices would improve immeasurably if they were guided by 'feminine' principles—qualities like love and care and intuition" (17).

27. Buchanan is traveling with Cynthia Brito, a photographer, who is prompting Paiakan in this dialogue.

28. Following Richard Parker's ethnographic research into new sexualities in contemporary Brazil, Roberto Reis has discussed the overlappings, in Brazilian colloquial usage, of "eating" and "having sex" within the Portuguese verb *comer.* "Sexual acts," he writes, "therefore establish a difference and a *radical heterogeneity* by just changing the individual into either the 'eater' or the 'eaten'" (105; my emphasis). Meanwhile, Fatimah Tobing Rony has observed a similar parallel established through the imaging of race as image of desire within the ethnographic. She writes about Martin Johnson's 1917 film *Cannibals of the South Seas:* "In this film, a sensational narrative of cannibalism and rape is spun out of a rather innocuous image of a man staring at the camera. There is nothing in the man's face or actions to suggest that he is a cannibal: the spectacle is

constructed entirely out of text. The Johnsons speak for the natives' desire, but what is revealed is their own fear, their own fascinating cannibalism, and consequently the audience's fearful delight in confronting the gaze of the 'cannibal'" (89–90).

29. In a 29 November 1994 article in the *New York Times* we read, "A judge in Redencão, a city in the state of Pará, said there was no evidence to support the charge by an 18-year-old woman that she had been raped and tortured by Chief Paulinio Paiakan in May 1992. The Judge, Elder Lisboa Ferreira da Costa, said that Mr. Paiakan's wife, Irekan (*sic*), had carried out an attack on the woman. Under Brazilian law, however, she cannot be prosecuted because she does not speak Portuguese and is not considered acculturated" (A10). I thank Barbara Price for bringing the story of Paiakan's acquittal to my attention.

Works Cited

Alarcón, Norma. "*Tradductora, Traditora:* A Paradigmatic Figure of Chicana Feminism." In *Dangerous Liaisons: Gender, Nation, and Postcolonial Perspectives.* Minneapolis: University of Minnesota Press, 1997.

Allen, Elizabeth. "Brazil: Indians and the New Constitution." *Third World Quarterly* 11: 4 (October 1989): 148–65.

Anzaldúa, Gloria. *Borderlands/La Frontera: The New Mestiza.* San Francisco: Aunt Lute Books, 1987.

Appadurai, Arjun. "Disjuncture and Difference in the Global Cultural Economy." In *Colonial Discourse and Postcolonial Theory.* Ed. Patrick Williams and Laura Chrisman. New York: Columbia University Press, 1994.

Armstrong, Nancy. "The Rise of the Domestic Woman." In *Feminisms: An Anthology of Literary Theory and Criticism.* Ed. Robyn R. Warhol and Diane Price Herndl. New Brunswick, N.J.: Rutgers University Press, 1991.

Aronowitz, Stanley, Dawn Esposito, William DiFazio, and Margaret Yard. "The Post-Work Manifesto." In *Post-Work: The Wages of Cybernation.* Ed. Stanley Aronowitz and Jonathan Cutler. New York: Routledge, 1998.

Asch, Timothy, with Jesus Ignacio Dardozo, Hortensia Cabellero, and Jose Bortoli. "The Story We Now Want to Hear Is Not Ours to Tell: Relinquishing Control over Representation: Toward Sharing Visual Communication Skills with the Yanomami." *Visual Anthropology Review* 7: 2 (Fall 1991): 102–6.

Ashcraft, Bill, Gareth Griffiths, and Helen Tiffin. *The Empire Writes Back: Theory and Practice in Post-Colonial Literatures.* New York: Routledge, 1989.

Bamberger, Joan. "Exit and Voice in Central Brazil: The Politics of Flight in Kayapó Society." In *Dialectical Societies: The Gê and Bororo of Central Brazil.* Ed. David Maybury-Lewis. Cambridge: Harvard University Press, 1979.

———. "The Myth of Matriarchy: Why Men Rule in Primitive Society." In *Woman,*

Culture, and Society. Ed. Michelle Zimbalist Rosaldo and Louise Lamphere. Stanford: Stanford University Press, 1974.

Banks, James A. et al. *World: Adventures in Time and Place*. New York: Macmillan/McGraw-Hill, 1997.

Barkan, Elazar. "Victorian Promiscuity: Greek Ethics and Primitive Exemplars." In *Prehistories of the Future: The Primitivist Project and the Culture of Modernism*. Ed. Elazar Barkan and Ronald Bush. Stanford: Stanford University Press, 1995.

Barrett, Clark, and Robert R. Warner. "Female Influences on Male Reproductive Success." In *Feminism and Evolutionary Biology: Boundaries, Intersections, and Frontiers*. Ed. Patricia Adair Gowaty. New York: Chapman and Hall, 1997.

Barrig, Maruja. Personal interview, 26 July 1995.

———. "Pitucas y marocas en la nueva narrative peruana." *Hueso húmero* 9 (1981): 71–89.

Barthes, Roland. *Camera Lucida: Reflections on Photography*. Trans. Richard Howard. New York: Hill and Wang, 1981.

Bataille, Georges. *The Accursed Share: An Essay on General Economy*. Vols. 1 and 3. Trans. Robert Hurley. New York: Zone Books, 1993.

———. *Erotism: Death & Sensuality*. Trans. Mary Dalwood. San Francisco: City Lights Books, 1986.

Bederman, Gail. *Manliness and Civilization: A Cultural History of Gender and Race in the United States, 1880–1917*. Chicago: University of Chicago Press, 1995.

Beer, Gillian. *Darwin's Plots: Evolutionary Narrative in Darwin, George Eliot and Nineteenth-Century Fiction*. London: Routledge and Kegan Paul, 1983.

Béjar, Eduardo. "La fuga erótica de Mario Vargas Llosa." *Symposium* (Winter 1993): 243–56.

Benjamin, Walter. "The Work of Art in the Age of Mechanical Reproduction." *Illuminations: Essays and Reflections*. Ed. Hannah Arendt. Trans. Harry Zohn. New York: Schocken Books, 1968.

Bennett de Marrais, Kathleen, and Margaret D. LeCompte. *The Way Schools Work: A Sociological Analysis of Education*. 2d ed. White Plains, N.Y.: Longman, 1995.

Bhabha, Homi K. "The Other Question: The Stereotype and Colonial Discourse." In *The Sexual Subject: A* Screen *Reader in Sexuality*. New York: Routledge, 1992.

———. "Of Mimicry and Man: The Ambivalence of Colonial Discourse." *October: The First Decade*. Cambridge: Massachusetts Institute of Technology and *October* Magazine, 1987.

———. "Signs Taken for Wonders: Questions of Ambivalence and Authority under a Tree Outside of Delhi, May 1817." *Critical Inquiry* 12: 1 (1985): 144–65.

———. "Of Mimicry and Man: The Ambivalence of Colonial Discourse." *October* 28 (1984): 125–33.

Blondet, Cecilia M. *Las mujeres y el poder: Una historia de Villa El Salvador*. Lima: Instituto de Estudios Peruanos, 1991.

———. "Nuevas formas de hacer política: las amas de casa populares." In *El movimiento popular de mujeres como respuesta a la crisis*. Lima: Cendoc, 1991: 195–207.

Booker, M. Keith. *Vargas Llosa among the Postmodernists*. Gainesville: University Press of Florida, 1994.

Bravo, Victor. *Magias y maravillas el el continente literario: para un deslinde del realismo mágico y lo real maravilloso.* Caracas: La Casa de Bello, 1988.

"Brazilian Indian Acquitted in Rape Case." *New York Times,* 29 November 1994, A10.

Brennan, Timothy. "The National Longing for Form." *Nation and Narration.* New York: Routledge, 1990.

Breton, André. *Nadja.* Trans. Richard Howard. New York: Grove Press, 1960.

Brisebois, Debbie. "The Inuit Broadcasting Corporation." *Anthropologica* 25: 1 (1983): 107–15.

Buchanan, Rob. "The Rainforest Rape." *Details* (March 1993): 46–56.

Butler, Judith. *The Psychic Life of "Power": Theories in Subjection.* Stanford: Stanford University Press, 1997.

———. *Bodies That Matter: On the Discursive Limits of "Sex."* New York: Routledge, 1993.

———. *Gender Trouble: Feminism and the Subversion of Identity.* New York: Routledge, 1990.

Cabello de Carbonera, Mercedes. "Inflencia de la mujer en la civilización." *El Album* 19 (13 October 1874).

Canclini, Néstor García. *Hybrid Cultures: Strategies for Entering and Leaving Modernity.* Trans. Christopher L. Chiappari and Silvia L. López. Minneapolis: University of Minnesota Press, 1995.

Caplan, Jane. "Sexuality and Homosexuality." In *Women in Society: Interdisciplinary Essays.* Ed. Cambridge Women's Studies Group. London: Virago Press, 1981.

Carelli, Vincent. *The Spirit of TV.* Centro de Trabalho Indigenista, 1990.

Carneiro da Cunha, Manuela. *Os direitos do Indio: Ensaios e documentos.* São Paulo: Editora Brasiliense, 1987.

Carpentier, Alejo. "Conciencia e identidad de América." *Ensayos. Obras completas de Alejo Carpentier.* Vol. 13. Mexico City: Siglo Veintiuno, 1990.

———. "De lo real maravilloso americano." *Ensayos. Obras completas de Alejo Carpentier.* Vol. 13. Mexico City: Siglo Veintiuno, 1990.

———. "La cultura de los pueblos que habitan en las tierras del mar Caribe." *Ensayos. Obras completas de Alejo Carpentier.* Vol. 13. Mexico City: Siglo Veintiuno, 1990.

———. "Lo barroco y lo real maravilloso." *Ensayos. Obras completas de Alejo Carpentier.* Vol. 13. Mexico City: Siglo Veintiuno, 1990.

———. "Problemática del tiempo y el idioma en la moderna novela latinoamericana." *Ensayos. Obras completas de Alejo Carpentier.* Vol. 13. Mexico City: Siglo Veintiuno, 1990.

———. *Ecue-Yamba-O.* Madrid: Alianza Editorial, 1989.

———. *Explosion in a Cathedral.* Trans. John Sturrock. New York: Noonday Press, 1963.

———. *The Lost Steps.* Trans. Harriet de Onís. New York: Noonday Press, 1956.

Carter, Julian. "Normality, Whiteness, Authorship: Evolutionary Sexology and the Primitive Pervert." In *Science and Homosexualities.* Ed. Vernon A. Rosario. New York: Routledge, 1997.

Castle, Terry. *The Apparitional Lesbian: Female Homosexuality and Modern Culture.* New York: Columbia University Press, 1993.

Cawelti, John. *The Six-Gun Mystique.* 2d ed. Bowling Green, Ohio: Bowling Green State University Popular Press, 1984.

Chanady, Amaryll. "The Territorialization of the Imaginary in Latin America: Self-Affirmation and Resistance to Metropolitan Paradigms." In *Magical Realism: Theory, History, Community.* Ed. Lois Parkinson Zamora and Wendy B. Faris. Durham: Duke University Press, 1995.

Chauncey, George Jr. "From Sexual Inversion to Homosexuality: Medicine and the Changing Conceptualization of Female Deviance." *Salmagundi* 58/59 (Fall/Winter 1983): 114–46.

Chiampi, Irlemar. "Alejo Carpentier y el surrealismo." *Revista de La Universidad de México* 37: 5 (1981): 2–10.

Chomsky, Noam. *Profit over People: Neoliberalism and Global Order.* New York: Seven Stories Press, 1999.

Cixous, Hélène. *Reading with Clarice Lispector.* Ed. and trans. Verena Andermatt Conley. Minneapolis: University of Minnesota Press, 1990.

Clarke, Patricia. *The Governesses: Letters from the Colonies, 1862–1882.* London: Hutchinson, 1985.

Cockburn, Alexander. "Beat the Devil: The Lynching of Paulinho Paiakan." *The Nation* (28 September 1992): 314–15.

Colás, Santiago. "Of Creole Symptoms, Cuban Fantasies, and Other Latin American Postcolonial Ideologies." *PMLA* 110: 3 (May 1995): 382–96.

Conklin, Beth A. "Body Paint, Feathers, and VCRs: Aesthetics and Authenticity in Amazonian Activism." *American Ethnologist* 24: 4 (1997): 711–37.

———, and Laura R. Graham. "The Shifting Middle Ground: Amazonian Indians and Eco-Politics." *American Anthropologist* 97: 4 (1995): 695–710.

Conrad, Joseph. *An Outcast of the Islands.* London: Thomas Nelson, 1919.

———. *Chance: A Tale in Two Parts.* London: J. M. Dent, 1913.

———. *Almayer's Folly: A Story of an Eastern River. Last Essays.* London: Thomas Nelson, 1895.

Cooper, Marc. "George W.'s Straw Party: In Iowa, the GOP Gets a Makeover for 2000." *The Nation* (6–13 September 1999): 11–16.

Cornejo-Polar, Antonio. "Una heterogeneidad no dialéctica: Sujecto y discurso migrantes en el Perú moderno." *Revista Iberoamericana* 62: 176–77 (July–December 1996): 837–44.

Cox, C. B. *Joseph Conrad: The Modern Imagination.* London: J. M. Dent, 1974.

Cox, Larry. "In Brazil, Indians Start Fighting Back." *New York Times* (3 August 1992).

Da Cunha, Euclides. *Rebellion in the Backlands (Os sertões).* Trans. Samuel Putnam. Chicago: University of Chicago Press, 1944.

Darwin, Charles. *The Origin of Species: By Means of Natural Selection or the Preservation of Favored Races in the Struggle for Life.* New York: Modern Library, 1993.

———. *The Variation of Animals and Plants Under Domestication.* Vol. 2. New York: Appleton, 1897.

———. *The Descent of Man and Selection in Relation to Sex.* New York: Appleton, 1896.

Davin, Anna. "Imperialism and Motherhood." *History Workshop: A Journal of Socialist Historians* 5 (Spring 1978): 9–65.

Dawkins, Richard. *The Selfish Gene.* New York: Oxford University Press, 1976.

De Castro, Nella, Lourdes y Flores, and Beatriz y Merino. "Mesa Redonda: La participación de la mujer en el 90." *Libertad.* Vol. 2. Lima: Pro-Desarrollo, 1988.

De la Campa, Román. "Latinoamérica y sus nuevos cartógrafos: Discurso postcolonial, diásporas intelectuales y enunciación fronteriza." *Revista Iberoamericana* 62: 176–77 (July–December 1996): 697–717.

———. "On Latin Americanism and the Postcolonial Turn." *Canadian Review of Comparative Literature* 22: 3–4 (September–December 1995): 745–71.

De Soto, Hernando. *El otro Sendero: La revolución informal.* Lima: Instituto Libertad y Democracia, 1986.

Degler, Carl N. "Does Sex Tell Us Anything?" In *In Search of Human Nature: The Decline and Revival of Darwinism in American Social Thought.* New York: Oxford University Press, 1991.

———. "What Ought to Be and What Was Women's Sexuality in the Nineteenth Century." *American Historical Review* 79: 5 (December 1974): 1467–90.

Degregori, Carlos Ivan. *El aprendiz de brujo y el curandero chino.* Lima: Instituto de Estudios Peruanos, 1991.

Derrida, Jacques. *Of Grammatology.* Trans. Gayatri Chakrovorty Spivak. Reprint. Baltimore: The Johns Hopkins University Press, 1976.

Devi, Mahasweta. *Imaginary Maps.* Trans. Gayatri Chakravorty Spivak. New York: Routledge, 1995.

Diggs, Marylynne. "Surveying the Intersection: Pathology, Secrecy, and the Discourses of Racial and Sexual Identity." In *Critical Essays: Gay and Lesbian Writers of Color.* Ed. Emmanuel S. Nelson. New York: Haworth Press, 1993.

Dillon, Sam. "Celebrated Defender of the Amazon Fighting Controversial Rape Charge." *Miami Herald* (12 July 1992): 1.

Dirlik, Arif. "The Postcolonial Aura: Third World Criticism and the Age of Global Capitalism." In *Dangerous Liaisons: Gender, Nation, and Postcolonial Perspectives.* Ed. Anne McClintock, Aamir Mufti, and Ella Shohat. Minneapolis: University of Minnesota Press, 1997.

Dowden, Wilfred S. *Joseph Conrad: The Imaged Style.* Nashville: Vanderbilt University Press, 1970.

Ellis, Havelock. *Studies in the Psychology of Sex.* Vol. 2. New York: Random House, 1910.

———. *Studies in the Psychology of Sex.* Vol. 1. New York: Random House, 1901.

———. "Sexual Inversion in Women." *Alienist and Neurologist* 16 (1895): 141–58.

Faderman, Lillian. *Odd Girls and Twilight Lovers: A History of Lesbian Life in Twentieth-Century America.* New York: Penguin, 1991.

Fedigan, Linda Marie. "The Changing Role of Women in Models of Human Evolution." *Annual Review of Anthropology* 15 (1986): 25–66.

Feito, Patricia Maria. *Gender, Sexuality, and Authority in the Modern British Novel: Virginia Woolf's* Orlando, *E. M. Forster's* Maurice *and Joseph Conrad's* Chance. Ann Arbor: University of Michigan Press, 1991.

Ferguson, Brian. Personal interview, 15 April 1994.

Florez, Nélida. *La mujer en la novela de Mario Vargas Llosa.* Lima: 1993.

Flower, W. H. and James Murie. "Account of the Dissection of a Bushwoman." *Journal of Anatomy and Physiology* 17 (1867): 189–208.

Ford, Charles A. "Homosexual Practices of Institutionalized Females." *Journal of Abnormal and Social Psychiatry* 23 (January–March 1929): 442–48.

Foucault, Michel. *The History of Sexuality: An Introduction.* Vol. 1. Trans. Robert Hurley. New York: Vintage Books, 1978.

Franco, Jean. "Apuntes sobre la crítica feminista y la literatura hispanoamericana." *Hispanámerica* 15: 45 (1986): 31–43.

———. "Self-Destructing Heroines." *Minnesota Review* 22 (1984): 105–115.

Fraser, Gail. "Empire of the Senses: Miscegenation in *Outcast of the Islands.*" *Contexts for Conrad.* Ed. Keith Carabine, Owen Knowles, and Wieslaw Krajka. Lublin: Maria Curie-Sklodowska University, 1993.

Fraser, Nancy. Justice Interruptus: Critical Reflections on the "Postsocialist" Condition, New York: Routledge, 1997.

Freud, Sigmund. *A Phylogenetic Fantasy: Overview of the Transference Neuroses.* Ed. Ilse Grubrich-Simitis. Trans. Axel Hoffer and Peter T. Hoffer. Cambridge: Belknap Press/Harvard University Press, 1987.

———. "A Case of Paranoia Running Counter to the Psychoanalytic Theory of the Disease." *Sexuality and the Psychology of Love.* Ed. Philip Rieff. New York: Collier Books, 1963.

———. *Dora: An Analysis of a Case of Hysteria.* Ed. Philip Rieff. Trans. Mr. and Mrs. James Strachey. New York: Collier Books, 1963.

———. "Fetishism." *Sexuality and the Psychology of Love.* Ed. Philip Rieff. Trans. James Strachey. New York: Collier Books, 1963.

———. "The History of Infantile Neurosis." *Three Case Histories.* Ed. Philip Rieff. New York: Collier Books, 1963.

———. "On Narcissism: An Introduction." *General Psychological Theory.* Ed. Philip Rieff. New York: Collier Books, 1963.

———. "The Psychogenesis of a Case of Homosexuality in a Woman." *Sexuality and the Psychology of Love.* Ed. Philip Rieff. New York: Collier Books, 1963.

———. *Three Essays on the Theory of Sexuality.* Ed. and trans. James Strachey. New York: Basic Books, 1962.

———. *The Ego and the Id.* Ed. James Strachey. Trans. Joan Riviere. New York: W. W. Norton, 1960.

———. *Totem and Taboo: Some Points of Agreement between the Mental Lives of Savages and Neurotics.* Trans. James Strachey. New York: W. W. Norton, 1950.

Friedman, Thomas L. *The Lexus and the Olive Tree.* New York: Farrar, Straus and Giroux, 1999.

Fuentes, Carlos. *The Death of Artemio Cruz.* Trans. Sam Hileman. New York: Farrar, Straus and Giroux, 1964.

Fuss, Diana. *Identification Papers.* New York: Routledge, 1995.

———. "Freud's Fallen Women: Identification, Desire, and 'A Case of Homosexuality in a Woman.'" *Yale Journal of Criticism* 6: 1 (Spring 1993): 1–23.

———. *Essentially Speaking: Feminism, Nature and Difference.* New York: Routledge, 1989.

Gallop, Jane. *The Daughter's Seduction: Feminism and Psychoanalysis.* Ithaca: Cornell University Press, 1982.

García Canclini, Néstor. *Culturas híbridas: Estrategias para entrar y salir de la modernidad.* Mexico City: Editorial Grijalbo, 1989.

Gathorne-Hardy, Jonathan. *The Rise and Fall of the British Nanny.* London: Hodder and Stoughton, 1972.

Gikandi, Simon. *Maps of Englishness: Writing Identity in the Culture of Colonialism.* New York: Columbia University Press, 1996.

Gilbert, J. Allen. "Homo-sexuality and Its Treatment." *Journal of Nervous and Mental Disease* 52 (1920): 297–322.

Gilbert, Sandra M. "Rider Haggard's Heart of Darkness." *Partisan Review* 5: 3 (1983): 444–52.

———, and Susan Gubar. *No Man's Land: The Place of the Woman Writer in the Twentieth Century.* Vol. 2: *Sexchanges.* New Haven: Yale University Press, 1989.

Gillon, Adam. "*Under Western Eyes, Chance,* and *Victory*": *Joseph Conrad.* Ed. Harold Bloom. New York: Chelsea House, 1986.

Gilman, Sander L. *The Case of Sigmund Freud: Medecine and Identity at the Fin de Siècle.* Baltimore: Johns Hopkins University Press, 1993.

———. *Difference and Pathology: Stereotypes of Sexuality, Race, and Madness.* Ithaca: Cornell University Press, 1985.

Ginsburg, Faye. "Embedded Aesthetics: Creating a Discursive Space for Indigenous Media." *Cultural Anthropology* 9: 3 (1994): 365–82.

———. "Aboriginal Media and the Australian Imaginary." *Public Culture* 4: 3 (Spring 1993): 557–78.

———. "Indigenous Media: Faustian Contract or Global Village?" *Cultural Anthropology* 6: 1 (1991): 92–112.

———. "In Whose Image? Indigenous Media From Aboriginal Central Australia." *CVA Review* (1989–91): 16–20.

Giovannini, Arno. *Entre culturas:* Los pasos perdidos *de Alejo Carpentier.* Bern: Peter Lang, 1991.

Giroux, Henry A. "The Politics of National Identity and the Pedagogy of Multiculturalism in the USA." In *Multicultural States: Rethinking Difference and Identity.* Ed. David Bennett. New York: Routledge, 1998.

Gomes, Laurentino and Paulo Silber. "A explosão do instinto selvagem." *Veja* (10 June 1992): 68–73.

González Echevarría, Roberto. "Latin American and Comparative Literatures." In *Poetics of the Americas: Race, Founding, and Textuality.* Ed. Bainard Cowan and Jefferson Humphries. Baton Rouge: Louisiana State University Press, 1997.

———. *Celestina's Brood: Continuities of the Baroque in Spanish and Latin American Literatures.* Durham: Duke University Press, 1993.

———. Introducción to *Los pasos perdidos,* by Alejo Carpentier. Madrid: Letras Hispánicas, 1985.

———. *Alejo Carpentier: The Pilgrim at Home.* Ithaca: Cornell University Press, 1977.

González, Eduardo. "*Los pasos perdidos*: El Azar y la Aventura." *Revista Iberoamericana* 38: 81 (1972): 585–613.

Good, Kenneth. *Into the Heart: One Man's Pursuit of Love and Knowledge among the Yanomama.* New York: Simon and Schuster, 1991.

Gould, Stephen Jay. "Dorothy, It's Really Oz." *Time* (23 August 1999): 59.

———. *Ontogeny and Phylogeny.* Cambridge: Belknap Press/Harvard University Press, 1977.

Gregor, Thomas. *Anxious Pleasures: The Sexual Lives of an Amazonian People.* Chicago: University of Chicago Press, 1985.

Groneman, Carol. "Nymphomania: The Historical Construction of Female Sexuality." In *Deviant Bodies: Critical Perspectives on Difference in Science and Popular Culture.* Ed. Jennifer Terry and Jacqueline Urla. Bloomington: Indiana University Press, 1995.

Guy, Donna J. "'White Slavery,' Citizenship and Nationality in Argentina." In *Nationalisms and Sexualities.* Ed. Andrew Parker, Mary Russo, Doris Sommer, and Patricia Yaeger. New York: Routledge, 1992.

Haggard, Rider H. *She.* New York: Signet, 1994.

Hall, Stuart. "When Was 'the Post-colonial'? Thinking at the Limit." In *The Post-Colonial Question: Common Skies, Divided Horizons.* Ed. Iain Chambers and Lidia Curti. New York: Routledge, 1996.

Haraway, Donna J. *Simians, Cyborgs, and Women: The Reinvention of Nature.* New York: Routledge, 1991.

Harding, Sandra. "Women's Standpoints on Nature: What Makes Them Possible." *Osiris* 12 (1997): 186–200.

Hart, Lynda. *Fatal Women: Lesbian Sexuality and the Mark of Aggression.* Princeton: Princeton University Press, 1994.

Harvey, David. "What's Green and Makes the Environment Go Round?" In *The Cultures of Globalization.* Ed. Fredric Jameson and Masao Miyoshi. Durham: Duke University Press, 1998.

Herman, Edward S., and Robert W. McChesney. *The Global Media: The New Missionaries of Corporate Capitalism.* Washington, D.C.: Cassell, 1997.

Horkheimer, Max, and Theodor W. Adorno. *Dialectic of Enlightenment.* Trans. John Cumming. New York: Continuum, 1991.

Horn, David G. "This Norm Which Is Not One: Reading the Female Body in Lombroso's Anthropology." In *Deviant Bodies: Critical Perspectives on Difference in Science and Popular Culture.* Ed. Jennifer Terry and Jacqueline Urla. Bloomington: Indiana University Press, 1995.

Howard, William Lee. "Effeminate Men and Masculine Women." *New York Medical Journal* (1900): 686–87.

Hubbard, Ruth. *The Politics of Women's Biology.* New Brunswick, N.J.: Rutgers University Press, 1990.

Hughes, Kathryn. *The Victorian Governess.* London: Hambledon Press, 1993.

Hyam, Ronald. *Empire and Sexuality: The British Experience.* Manchester, Eng.: Manchester University Press, 1991.

Irigaray, Luce. *Speculum of the Other Woman.* Trans. Gillian C. Gill. Ithaca: Cornell University Press, 1985.

Jagose, Annamarie. *Lesbian Utopics.* New York: Routledge, 1994.

James, Henry. *The Turn of the Screw and Other Short Fiction.* New York: Bantam Books, 1983.

———. *The Bostonians.* New York: Signet, 1979.

Jameson, Fredric. "Notes on Globalization as a Philosophical Issue." In *The Cultures of Globalization.* Ed. Fredric Jameson and Masao Miyoshi. Durham: Duke University Press, 1998.

———. *The Political Unconscious: Narrative as a Socially Symbolic Act.* Ithaca: Cornell University Press, 1981.

JanMohamed, Abdul R. "Sexuality On/Of the Racial Border: Foucault, Wright, and the Articulation of 'Racialized Sexuality.'" In *Discourses of Sexuality: From Aristotle to AIDS.* Ed. Donna C. Stanton. Ann Arbor: University of Michigan Press, 1992.

Jaroff, Leon. "Iceman." *Time* (26 October 1992): 62–66.

Johnson, Joseph Taber. "On Some of the Apparent Peculiarities of Parturition in the Negro Race, With Remarks on Race and Pelves in General." *American Journal of Obstetrics and Diseases of Women and Children* 8 (1875): 88–123.

Johnson, Julie M. "The Damsel and Her Knights: The Goddess and the Grail in Conrad's *Chance.*" *Conradiana* 13: 3 (1981): 221–28.

Kadir, Djelal. *Questing Fictions: Latin America's Family Romance.* Minneapolis: University of Minnesota Press, 1986.

Kazin, Alfred. Introduction to *Chance*, by Joseph Conrad. New York: Signet, 1992.

Keating, AnnLouise. "Myth Smashers, Myth Makers: (Re)Visionary Techniques in the Works of Paula Gunn Allen, Gloria Anzaldúa, and Audre Lorde." In *Critical Essays: Gay and Lesbian Writers of Color.* Ed. Emmanuel S. Nelson. New York: Harrington Park Press, 1993.

Kiernan, Jas. G. "Psychological Aspects of the Sexual Appetite." *Alienist and Neurologist* 12 (1891): 188–219.

Klor de Alva, J. Jorge. "The Postcolonialization of the (Latin) American Experience: A Reconsideration of 'Colonialism,' 'Postcolonialism,' and 'Mestizaje.'" In *After Colonialism: Imperial Histories and Postcolonial Displacements.* Princeton: Princeton University Press, 1995.

———. "Colonialism and Postcolonialism as (Latin) American Mirages." *Colonial Latin American Review* 1: 1–2 (1992): 3–23.

Kovel, Joel. "Dispatches from the Science Wars." *Science Wars.* Ed. Andrew Ross. Durham: Duke University Press, 1996.

Krasner, James. *The Entangled Eye: Visual Perception and the Representation of Nature in Post-Darwinian Narrative.* New York: Oxford University Press, 1992.

Kutzinski, Vera M. *Sugar's Secrets: Race and the Erotics of Cuban Nationalism.* Charlottesville: University Press of Virginia, 1993.

Laqueur, Thomas. *Making Sex: Body and Gender from the Greeks to Freud.* Cambridge: Harvard University Press, 1990.

Lemonick, Michael D., and Andrea Dorfman. "Up from the Apes: Remarkable New Evicence Is Filling in the Story of How We Became Human." *Time* (23 August 1999): 50–58.

Levine, George. *Darwin and the Novelists: Patterns of Science in Victorian Fiction.* Chicago: University of Chicago Press, 1988.

Lightman, Bernard. Introduction to *Victorian Science in Context.* Chicago: University of Chicago Press, 1997.

Lindon, Eugene. "Can Animals Think?" *Time* (6 September 1999): 56–60.

Lispector, Clarice. *The Hour of the Star.* Trans. Giovanni Pontiero. New York: New Directions, 1986.

Lloyd, Elisabeth A. "Pre-Theoretical Assumptions in Evolutionary Explanations of Female Sexuality." *Feminism and Science.* Ed. Evelyn Fox Keller and Helen E. Longino. New York: Oxford University Press, 1996.

Lombroso, Caesar, and William Ferrero. *The Female Offender.* New York: Appleton, 1915.

Lyell, Charles. "Principles of Geology, 1830–1833." In *Darwin: Texts, Backgrounds, Contemporary Opinion, Critical Essays.* Ed. Philip Appleman. New York: W. W. Norton, 1970.

MacDonald, Ian R. "Magical Eclecticism: *Los pasos perdidos* and Jean-Paul Sartre." *Forum for Modern Language Studies* 15: 2 (April 1979): 97–113.

Macera, Pablo. "Sexo y coloniaje." In *Trabajos de historia.* Vol. 3. Lima: Instituto Nacional de Cultura, 1977.

Mariátegui, José Carlos. *Seven Interpretive Essays on Peruvian Reality.* Trans. Marjory Urquidi. Austin: University of Texas Press, 1971.

Martí, José. "Nuestra América." *Política de nuestra América.* Mexico City: Siglo Veintiuno, 1987.

———. "Our America." *Our America by José Martí: Writings on Latin America and the Struggle for Cuban Independence.* Ed. Philip S. Foner. Trans. Elinor Randall. New York: Monthly Review Press, 1977.

McCallum, Cecilia. "Ritual and the Origin of Sexuality in the Alto Xingo." *Sex and Violence.* Ed. Penelope Harvey and Peter Gow. New York: Routledge, 1994.

———. "*Veja* Magazine's Payakan: The Image of the Indian in Brazilian Culture." Paper presented to the symposium "Discovering Native America: Images, Text, Politics" at the Third International Festival of Ethnographic Film, 14–19 September 1992.

McClintock, Anne. *Imperial Leather: Race, Gender and Sexuality in the Colonial Contest.* New York: Routledge, 1995.

McCracken, Scott. "Postmodernism, a *Chance* to Rearead?" *Cultural Politics at the Fin de Siècle.* Ed. Scott McCracken and Sally Ledger. Cambridge: Cambridge University Press, 1995.

Meyer, Bernard C. *Joseph Conrad: A Psychoanalytic Biography.* Princeton: Princeton University Press, 1967.

Michaels, Julia. "Rape Trial Highlights Brazilian Native Rights." *Christian Science Monitor* (19 June 1992).

Milner, Richard. "Attack of the Sea Tiger." *Natural History* (January 1995): 65.

Moffett, Matt. "Kayapo Indians Lose Their 'Green' Image." *Wall Street Journal* (29 December 1994): A6.

Mohanty, Chandra Talpade. "Women Workers and Capitalist Scripts: Ideologies of Domination, Common Interests, and the Politics of Solidarity." In *Feminist Genealogies, Colonial Legacies, Democratic Futures.* Ed. M. Jacqui Alexander and Chandra T. Mohanty. New York: Routledge, 1997.

Molloy, Sylvia. "Too Wilde for Comfort: Desire and Ideology In Fin-de-Siècle Spanish America." In *¿Entiendes?: Queer Readings, Hispanic Writings.* Ed. Emilie L. Bergmann and Paul Julian Smith. Durham: Duke University Press, 1995.

Montero, Oscar. "Notes for a Queer Reading of Latin American Literature." In *Queer Representations: Reading Lives, Reading Cultures.* Ed. Martin Duberman. New York: New York University Press, 1997.

Moore, Rachel. "Marketing Alterity." *Visual Anthropology Review* 8: 2 (Fall 1992): 16–26.

Mörner, Maguns. *Race Mixture in the History of Latin America.* Boston: Little, Brown, 1967.

Morris, Robert T. "Is Evolution Trying To Do Away with the Clitoris?" *Transactions of American Association of Obstetricians and Gynecologists* 5 (1892): 288–302.

Moscucci, Ornella. *The Science of Woman: Gynaecology and Gender in England, 1800–1929.* Cambridge: Cambridge University Press, 1990.

Mosedale, Susan Sleeth. "Science Corrupted: Victorian Biologists Consider 'The Woman Question.'" *Journal of the History of Biology* 11: 1 (1978): 3–55.

Müller-Bergh, Klaus. "Corrientes vanguardistas y surrealismo en la obra de Alejo Carpentier." *Revista hispánica moderna* 35 (1969): 323–40.

Mulvey, Laura. "Pandora: Topographies of the Mask and Curiosity." *Sexuality and Space.* Princeton: Princeton Architectural Press, 1992.

———. "Visual Pleasure and Narrative Cinema." *Screen* 16: 3 (Autumn 1975): 6–18.

Nadelhaft, Ruth. *Joseph Conrad: Feminist Readings.* Atlantic Highlands, N.J.: Humanities Press International, 1991.

———. "Women as Moral and Political Alternatives in Conrad's Early Novels." In *Joseph Conrad.* Ed. Harold Bloom. New York: Chelsea House, 1986.

Nietzsche, Friedrich. *On the Genealogy of Morals.* Trans. Walter Kaufmann and R. J. Hollingdale. New York: Vintage Books, 1967.

Norris, Margot. *Beasts of the Modern Imagination: Darwin, Nietzsche, Kafka, Ernst, and Lawrence.* Baltimore: Johns Hopkins University Press, 1985.

"O fim do romantismo: O roqueiro Sting descobriu que os índios adoram dinheiro e são pouco confiáveis." *Veja* (28 April 1993): 74–75.

Oliart, Patricia. "Temidos y despreciados: raza y género en la representación de las clases populares limeñas en la literatura del siglo XIX." In *Otras pieles: Género, historia y cultura.* Ed. Maruja Barrig y Narda Henríquez. Lima: Pontificia Universidad Católica del Perú, 1994.

Ortega, Julia. "El otro Vargas Llosa." *Postdata* 1 (December 1973): 21–24.

Otis, Margaret. "A Perversion Not Commonly Noted." *Journal of Abnormal Psychology* 8: 2 (June–July 1913): 113–16.

Oviedo, José Miguel. *Mario Vargas Llosa: La invención de una realidad.* 2d ed. Barcelona: Barral Editores, 1977.

Palmer, David Scott. "History, Politics, and Shining Path in Peru." Introduction to *Shining Path of Peru.* 2d ed. New York: St. Martin's Press, 1994.

Parker, Richard. *Bodies, Pleasures, and Passions.* Boston: Beacon Press, 1991.

Paz, Octavio. *The Labyrinth of Solitude.* Trans. Lysander Kemp, Yara Milos, and Rachel Phillips Belash. New York: Grove Press, 1985.

Pereira Coelho, Maria Claudia. "Rituals, Scandals, and Sex Crimes: Attempted Rape-Murders Across Two Generations." In *The Brazilian Puzzle: Culture on the Borderlands of the Western World.* Ed. David J. Hess and Roberto A. DaMatta. New York: Columbia University Press, 1995.

Perilli, Carmen. "Imágenes de la mujer en Carpentier y García Márquez: Mitificación y demitificación." Ph.D. diss., Universidad Nacional de Tucuman en Argentina, 1989.

Poisey, David, and William Hansen. *Starting Fire with Gunpowder.* 1991.

Pollard, Simon. "Samurai Spiders." *Natural History* (March 1995): 44–47.

Pollitt, Katha. "Weird Science." *The Nation* (20 September 1999): 10.

Poole, Deborah A. "A One-Eyed Gaze: Gender in 19th Century Illustration of Peru." *Dialectical Anthropology* 13 (1988): 333–54.

Poovey, Mary. *Uneven Developments: The Ideological Work of Gender in Mid-Victorian England.* Chicago: University of Chicago Press, 1988.

Posey, Daryl A. E-mail interview, 19–25 August 1996.

Pratt, Mary Louise. *Imperial Eyes: Travel Writing and Transculturation.* New York: Routledge, 1992.

Preston, Julia. "Brazilian Case Spurs Debate on Indians." *Washington Post* (17 August 1992).

Raiskin, Judith. "Inverts and Hyrids: Lesbian Rewritings of Sexual and Racial Identities." In *The Lesbian Postmodern.* Ed. Laura Doan. New York: Columbia University Press, 1994.

Rama, Angel. *The Lettered City.* Ed. and trans. John Charles Chasteen. Durham: Duke University Press, 1996.

Rayner, Jay. "The Mystery of the Disappearing Sperm." *Hot Air* 57 (April–June 1997): 15–16.

Reis, Roberto. "Representations of Family and Sexuality in Brazilian Cultural Discourse." Trans. Dário Borim and Ann Fifield-Borim. In *Bodies and Biases: Sexualities in Hispanic Cultures and Literatures.* Ed. David William Foster and Roberto Reis. Minneapolis: University of Minnesota Press, 1996.

Renton, Alice. *Tyrant or Victim?: A History of the British Nanny.* London: Weidenfeld and Nicolson, 1991.

Retamar, Roberto Fernández. *Calibán: Apuntes sobre la cultura de nuestra América.* Mexico City: Editorial Diogenes, 1972.

Richards, Evelleen. "Darwin and the Descent of Woman." *The Wider Domain of Evolutionary Thought.* Ed. David Oldroyd and Ian Langham. Boston: D. Reidel Publishing, 1983.

Rieselback, Helen Funck. *Conrad's Rebels: The Psychology of Revolution in the Novels from* Nostromo *to* Victory. Ann Arbor: University of Michigan Press, 1981.

Ritvo, Harriet. "Barring the Cross: Miscegenation and Purity in Eighteenth- and Nineteenth-Century Britain." *Human, All Too Human.* Ed. Diana Fuss. New York: Routledge, 1996.

Ritvo, Lucille B. "Carl Claus as Freud's Professor of the New Darwinian Biology." *International Journal of Psycho-Analysis* 53 (1972): 277–83.

———. "Darwin as the Source of Freud's Neo-Lamarckianism." *Journal of the American Psychoanalytic Association* 13: 3 (July 1965): 499–517.

Rivera, Eustasio. *La vorágine.* Guatemala: Editorial Piedra Santa, 1981.

Roddick, Anita. *Body and Soul: Profits With Principles—The Amazing Success Story of Anita Roddick and The Body Shop.* New York: Crown, 1991.

Rodríguez Ichaso, Mari. "Entrevista." *Vanidades Continental* (24 December 1985): 16–17.
Rojas-Paiewonsky, Lourdes. *Dos formas complentaria de mitificación y desmitificación de la mujer en la primera generación superrealista:* La creación *de Agustín Yáñez, y* Los pasos perdidos *de Alejo Carpentier.* Ann Arbor: University of Michigan Press, 1986.
Romanes, George John. "Mental Difference between Men and Women." In *Essays.* Ed. C. Lloyd Morgan. London: Longmans, Green, 1897.
Romeu, Raquel. "De la ciudad a la selva: Constantes y variables entre *Los pasos perdidos* y *El hablador.*" *Literatura del mundo hispánico.* Quito: Universidad San Francisco de Quito, Instituto Literario Cultural Hispánico, 1992.
Rony, Fatimah Tobing. *The Third Eye: Race, Cinema, and Ethnographic Spectacle.* Durham: Duke University Press, 1996.
Roof, Judith. *Reproductions of Reproduction: Imaging Symbolic Change.* New York: Routledge, 1996.
Ross, Andrew. "The Chicago Gangster Theory of Life." *Social Text* 35 (Summer 1993): 93–112.
Russett, Cynthia Eagle. *Sexual Science: The Victorian Construction of Womanhood.* Cambridge: Harvard University Press, 1991.
Said, Edward. *Joseph Conrad and the Fiction of Autobiography.* Cambridge: Harvard University Press, 1966.
Saleeby, C. W. *Woman and Womanhood: A Search for Principles.* New York: Mitchell Kennerley, 1911.
Sanger, Margaret. *Woman and the New Race.* New York: Brentano's, 1920.
Sarduy, Severo. *Barroco.* Buenos Aires: Editorial Sudamericana, 1974.
"The Savage Can Also Be Ignoble." *The Economist* (12 June 1993): 54.
Schabas, Margaret. "Victorian Economics and the Science of Mind." In *Victorian Science in Context.* Ed. Bernard Lightman. Chicago: University of Chicago Press, 1997.
Schatz, Thomas. *Hollywood Genres: Formulas, Filmmaking, and the Studio System.* New York: McGraw-Hill, 1981.
Schiebinger, Londa. *Nature's Body: Gender in the Making of Modern Science.* Boston: Beacon Press, 1993.
———. "Skeletons in the Closet: The First Illustrations of the Female Skeleton in Eighteenth-Century Anatomy." *Representations* 14 (1986): 44–82.
Schneebaum, Tobias. *Keep the River on Your Right.* New York: Grove Press, 1969.
Sharpe, Jenny. *Allegories of Empire: The Figure of Woman in the Colonial Text.* Minneapolis: University of Minnesota Press, 1993.
Shohat, Ella. "Notes on the 'Post-Colonial.'" *Social Text* 31–32 (1992): 99–113.
———. "The Struggle over Representation: Casting, Coalitions, and the Politics of Identification." In *Late Imperial Culture.* Ed. Román de la Campa, E. Ann Kaplan, and Michael Sprinker. New York: Verso, 1995.
Showalter, Elaine. *Sexual Anarchy: Gender and Culture at the Fin de Siècle.* New York: Viking, 1990.
Siegle, Robert. "The Two Texts of *Chance.*" *Conradiana* 16: 2 (1984): 83–101.
Silverstein, Ken. "Words from Our Sponsor." *The Nation* (22 March 1999): 7.

Skidmore, Thomas E. *Black into White: Race and Nationality in Brazilian Thought.* Durham: Duke University Press, 1993.

Slocum, Sally. "Woman the Gatherer: Male Bias in Anthropology." In *Toward an Anthropology of Women.* Ed. Rayna Reiter. New York: Monthly Review Press, 1975.

Smith-Rosenberg, Carroll. "Discourses of Sexuality and Subjectivity: The New Woman, 1870–1936." *Hidden from History: Reclaiming the Gay and Lesbian Past.* Ed. Martin Duberman, Martha Vicinus, and George Chauncey, Jr. New York: New American Library, 1989.

———, and Charles Rosenberg. "The Female Animal: Medical and Biological Views of Woman and Her Role in Nineteenth Century America." *Journal of American History* 60 (1973): 332–56.

Somerville, Siobhan. "Scientific Racism and the Emergence of the Homosexual Body." *Journal of the History of Sexuality* 5: 2 (October 1994): 243–66.

Sommer, Doris. *Foundational Fictions: The National Romances of Latin America.* Berkeley: University of California Press, 1991.

Soper, Kate. "Nature/'nature'" *FutureNatural: Nature, Science, Culture.* Ed. George Robertson, et al. New York: Routledge, 1996.

Sperling, Susan. "Baboons with Briefcases vs. Langurs in Lipstick: Feminism and Functionalism in Primate Studies." *Gender at the Crossroads of Knowledge: Feminist Anthropology in the Postmodern Era.* Ed. Micaela di Leonardo. Berkeley: University of California Press, 1991.

Spivak, Gayatri Chakravorty. *The Post-Colonial Critic: Interviews, Strategies, Dialogues.* New York: Routledge, 1990.

Stam, Robert. "Eurocentrism, Polycentrism, and Multicultural Pedagogy: Film and the Quincentennial." In *Late Imperial Culture.* Ed. Román de la Campa, E. Ann Kaplan, and Michael Sprinker. New York: Verso, 1995.

Stocking, George Jr. "The Persistence of Polygenist Thought in Post-Darwinian Anthropology." In *Race, Culture, and Evolution: Essays in the History of Anthropology.* New York: Free Press, 1968.

Stokes, Susan C. *Cultures in Conflict: Social Movements and the State in Peru.* Berkeley: University of California Press, 1995.

Stolcke, Verena. "Conquered Women." *NACLA Report on the Americas* 24: 5 (February 1991): 23–28.

———. *Marriage, Class and Colour in Nineteenth-Century Cuba: A Study of Racial Attitudes and Sexual Values in a Slave Society.* Ann Arbor: University of Michigan Press, 1989.

Stoler, Ann Laura. *Race and the Education of Desire: Foucault's* History of Sexuality *and the Colonial Order of Things.* Durham: Duke University Press, 1995.

———. "Carnal Knowledge and Imperial Power: Gender, Race, and Morality in Colonial Asia." *Gender at the Crossroads of Knowledge: Feminist Anthropology in the Postmodern Era.* Ed. Micaela di Leonardo. Berkeley: University of California Press, 1991.

"Subversion by Cassette." *Time* (11 September 1989): 80.

Suleri, Sara. "Woman Skin Deep: Feminism and the Postcolonial Condition." In *Colonial Discourse and Post-Colonial Theory: A Reader.* Ed. Patrick Williams and Laura Chrisman. New York: Columbia University Press, 1994.

Sulloway, Frank J. *Freud, Biologist of the Mind: Beyond the Psychoanalytic Legend.* New York: Basic Books, 1979.

Swann, Jim. "*Mater* and Nannie: Freud's Two Mothers and the Discovery of the Oedipus Complex." *American Imago* 31: 1 (Spring 1974): 1–64.

Tanner, Nancy, and Adrienne Zihlman. "Women in Evolution. Part II: Subsistence and Social Organization among Early Hominids." *Signs* 4: 1 (Autumn 1978): 4–20.

———. "Women in Evolution. Part I: Innovation and Selection in Human Origins." *Signs* 1: 3 (1976): 585–608.

Taussig, Michael. *Mimesis and Alterity: A Particular History of the Senses.* New York: Routledge, 1993.

Terry, Jennifer. "Anxious Slippages between 'Us' and 'Them': A Brief History of the Scientific Search for Homosexual Bodies." In *Deviant Bodies: Critical Perspectives on Difference in Science and Popular Culture.* Ed. Jennifer Terry and Jacqueline Urla. Bloomington: Indiana University Press, 1995.

Thomas, Julian. "The Mystery of the Missing Penis." *Science* (8 March 1997): 19.

Tompkins, Jame. *West of Everything: The Inner Life of Westerns.* New York: Oxford University Press, 1992.

Torgovnick, Marianna. *Gone Primitive: Savage Intellects, Modern Lives.* Chicago: University of Chicago Press, 1990.

Torres-Rosado, Santos. "La mujer como referente estético-literario en *El reino de este mundo* de Alejo Carpentier." *Cincinnati Romance Review* 10 (1991): 208–216.

Travis, Jennifer. "Clits in Court: *Salome*, Sodomy, and the Lesbian 'Sadist.'" In *Lesbian Erotics.* Ed. Karla Jay. New York: New York University Press, 1995.

Tschofen, Monique Y. "Post-Colonial Allegory and the Empire of Rape." *Canadian Review of Comparative Literature* 22: 3–4 (September–December 1995): 501–515.

Turner, Terence. "Social Body and Embodied Subject: Bodiliness, Subjectivity, and Sociality among the Kayapo." *Cultural Anthropology* 10: 2 (May 1995): 143–70.

———. Telephone interview with the author, 9 April 1994, and 13 July 1994.

———. "Representing, Resisting, Rethinking: Historical Transformations of Kayapo Culture and Anthropological Consciousness." In *Colonial Situations: Essays on the Contextualization of Ethnographic Knowledge.* Ed. George W. Stocking, Jr. Madison: University of Wisconsin Press, 1991.

———. "The Social Dynamics of Video Media in an Indigenous Society: The Cultural Meaning and the Personal Politics of Video-making in Kayapo Communities." *Visual Anthropology Review* 7: 2 (Fall 1991): 68–76.

———. "Visual Media, Cultural Politics and Anthropological Practice." *The Independent* (January–February 1991): 34–40.

———. *The Kayapo out of the Forest.* Granada Television, 1989.

———. *The Kayapo.* Granada Television, 1987.

———. "Kinship, Household, and Community Structure Among the Kayapó." In *Dialectical Societies: The Gê and Bororo of Central Brazil.* Ed. David Maybury-Lewis. Cambridge: Harvard University Press, 1979.

———, and Centro de Trabalho Indigenista (CTI). *Peace between Chiefs.* Directed by Mokuka Kaiapó. 1990.

Vargas Llosa, Mario. "La cultura en el ginceceo." Washington, D.C. April 1994.

———. *A Fish in the Water: A Memoir.* Trans. Helen Lane. New York: Penguin Books, 1994.
———. *Pantaleón y las visitadoras.* Reprint. Barcelona: Editorial Seix Barral, 1993.
———. *Acción para el cambio: El programa de gobierno del Frente Democrático.* Lima: Instituto Peruano de Administración de Empresas, 1989.
———. "Bataille o El rescate del Mal." In *Contra viento y marea.* Vol. 2: 1972–1983. Barcelona: Editorial Seix Barral, 1983, 1986.
———. "La cultura de la libertad." In *Contra viento y marea.* Vol. 2: 1972–1983. Barcelona: Editorial Seix Barral, 1983, 1986.
———. Prologue to *El otro sendero: la revolución informal,* by Hernando de Soto. Lima: Instituto Libertad y Democracia, 1986.
———. *The War of the End of the World.* Trans. Helen R. Lane. New York: Farrar, Straus and Giroux, 1984.
———. "La literatura es fuego." In *Contra viento y marea, 1962–82.* Barcelona: Editorial Seix Barral, 1983.
———. *La orgía perpetua.* Barcelona: Bruguera, 1978.
———. *García Márquez: historia de un deicidio.* Barcelona: Barral Editores, 1971.
Viana, Francisco. "Indio gente fina: Os caciques brasileiros que enriqueceram explorando como bons capitalistas as riquezas de suas reservas." *Isto É* (1 July 1992): 38–41.
Vidal, Hernán. "The Concept of Colonial and Postcolonial Discourse: A Perspective from Literary Criticism." *Latin American Research Review* 28: 3 (1993): 113–19.
Villar Márquez, Eliana. *Por mérito propio: mujer y política.* Lima: Flora Tristán, 1994.
Villavicencio, Maritza. *Del silencio a la palabra: Mujeres peruanas en los siglos XIX–XX.* Lima: Flora Tristán, 1992.
Wallace, Scott. "Rape and Politics in the Rain Forest." *Penthouse* (November 1993): 102–149.
Watson, Paul J. "Dancing in the Dome." *Natural History* (March 1995): 40–43.
Weatherford, Elizabeth. "Native Visions: The Growth of Indigenous Media." *Aperture* 119 (1990): 58–61.
Weeks, Jeffrey. "Havelock Ellis and the Politics of Sex Reform." In *Socialism and the New Life: The Personal and Sexual Politics of Edward Carpenter and Havelock Ellis.* Ed. Sheila Rowbotham and Jeffrey Weeks. London: Pluto Press, 1977.
Whittemore, Hank. "A Man Who Would Save the World." *Parade* (12 April 1992): 4–7.
Williams, Raymond Leslie. *Mario Vargas Llosa.* New York: Ungar, 1986.
Wright, Will. *Six Guns and Society: A Structural Study of the Western.* Berkeley: University of California Press, 1975.
Yarbro-Bejarano, Yvonne. "Chicana Literature from a Chicana Feminist Perspective." In *Feminisms: An Anthology of Literary Theory and Criticism.* Ed. Robyn R. Warhol and Diane Price Herndl. New Brunswick, N.J.: Rutgers University Press, 1993.
Yeazell, Ruth Bernard. "Nature's Courtship Plot in Darwin and Ellis." *Yale Journal of Criticism* 2: 2 (Spring 1989): 33–53.
Young, Robert J. C. *Colonial Desire: Hybridity in Theory, Culture and Race.* New York: Routledge, 1995.
Yúdice, George. "We Are *Not* the World." *Social Text* 31–32 (1992): 202–216.

Zamora, Lois Parkinson. "Magic Ruins/Magical Realism: Alejo Carpentier, François de Nomé, and the New World Baroque." In *Poetics of the Americas: Race, Founding, and Textuality.* Baton Rouge: Louisiana State University Press, 1997.

Zihlman, Adrienne L. "The Paleolithic Glass Ceiling: Women in Human Evolution." In *Women in Human Evolution.* Ed. Lori D. Hager. New York: Routledge, 1997.

———. "Misreading Darwin on Reproduction: Reductionism in Evolutionary Theory." In *Conceiving the New World Order: The Global Politics of Reproduction.* Ed. Faye Ginsburg and Rayna Rapp. Berkeley: University of California Press, 1995.

Zimmerman, Jonathan. "Relatively Speaking." *The New Republic* (6 September 1999): 13–14.

Zola, Emile. *Nana.* Trans. George Holden. New York: Penguin Books, 1972.

Robin Truth Goodman lives in New York City and has taught extensively in the City University of New York system. She has been a visiting assistant professor of women's and gender studies at the College of New Jersey and visiting scholar in women's studies at the University of New Mexico. She has also taught literature in La Paz, Bolivia, and Cuzco, Peru.

Index